THE DIETITIAN'S DILEMMA:

WHAT WOULD YOU DO IF YOUR HEALTH WAS RESTORED BY DOING THE OPPOSITE OF EVERYTHING YOU WERE TAUGHT?

Written by Michelle Hurn, Registered and Licensed Dietitian, Ultra Runner

Foreword by Dr. Nevada Gray PharmD, R.N.

Graphics by Health Coach Kait

Pictures, charts, artistic design by Ash Davis

Cover Photo by Corene Elia

Acknowledgments

To Mom and Dre, thank you for never giving up on me. Mom, I am so proud of everything you have overcome.

To my sisters, Heather, Kristen, and Stephanie, you guys are my heart.

To Meg Chatham, your friendship and guidance on how the heck to write a book has been life changing. I'm so grateful.

To Nevada Grey, the greatest friend and mentor one could ask for. Thank you for your support, for pushing me to keep going, and for sharing in my joy.

To all the members of the low-carbohydrate, ketogenic, and animal-nutrition based community who contributed their testimonies and have shown unwavering support for me and my endeavors. This book exists because of you guys.

To Corene Elia, the love of my life. I promise I'll take you on a nice vacation... someday. ☺

Table of Contents:

Introduction

What would you do if your health was restored by doing the opposite of everything you were taught?

If you are like most of the patients I met during my 11 years working in health care, you've tried every diet under the sun. Most men and women I saw in the acute care setting told me stories about meticulously counting calories, eating whole grains and vegetables religiously, exercising daily, and yet they were still finding they could not lose weight or make any improvements to their chronic conditions.

Our health care system has a narrative indicating that individuals who find themselves diabetic, obese, struggling with depression, or diseases of inflammation simply need to follow the nutrition guidelines, eat less, and move more.

I found that many of individuals I saw who were diagnosed with chronic conditions were doing just that: attempting to eat healthy and move as they were able. Unfortunately, they continued to be sick, obese, to suffer with debilitating depression, develop widespread, systemic infections, or end up with organ failure such as kidney failure or heart disease.

What's worse is that there is so much conflicting information available. A quick Google search of "healthy diet" will likely lead one down a rabbit hole of various theories of what humans *should* eat to thrive. Unfortunately, many of these ideals are motivated by corporate (profit-based) interests and have very little to do with restoring and maintaining health.

If you or someone you love has lost and gained hundreds of pounds on various diets, is overweight, diabetic, suffers low energy, poor sleep, feels hungry all the time, has frequent bouts of anxiety or depression, deals with gastrointestinal disorders such as Irritable Bowel Syndrome (IBS), ulcerative colitis, or frequent gas and bloating, has been diagnosed with hypertension, has chronic inflammation or an autoimmune disorder, or is in the depths or an eating disorder, I am here to offer a message and a different narrative than you have likely heard before.

This is not your fault. You do not lack willpower and you are not a moral failure. The fact that your mother, father, or entire lineage was diagnosed with a particular disease, such as diabetes, does not mean *you have to succumb to the same fate.*

Instead of blaming ourselves, I believe we need to look at our current national nutrition guidelines and entire health care system. Is it possible that we have been given incorrect, erroneous information about what humans need to eat to have vibrant physical and mental health?

Make no mistake, humans can survive eating all kinds of things. There are articles on individuals losing weight eating only chicken nuggets or Twinkies. Most individuals want not only to lose weight; they want food freedom. They want to eat in a way where they feel nourished, satiated, and will no longer need to worry about gaining weight or suffering from a debilitating illness. They would also like to experience feelings of calm and joy, while having the energy to pursue endeavors they feel passionate about.

If health could be restored quickly with minimal to zero side effects, could I continue to practice in a system that refused to allow me to teach this potentially lifesaving information?

I had a dilemma and a choice to make. I chose to speak out. In the following pages you will learn about my story. We will walk through various chronic diseases and we will unpack how the nutrition guidelines were developed. I will ask tough questions and I will empower you with my clinical experience, testimonies, and clinical trials. It is my sincerest hope that all of you find this information useful, inspiring, and that you make the choice to take your health back. It is within your reach; let me show you how.

Foreword

Over the past 100 years, medical science has advanced to teach us two valuable lessons: we are not merely victims of our genetic destiny, and our lifestyle choices matter. The USDA Dietary Guidelines persist in current practice as a "one size fits all" nutrition strategy, despite emerging evidence that low-carbohydrate nutrition approaches may prevent and even reverse metabolic illnesses like diabetes and obesity. Thus, enters The Dietitian's Dilemma.

Many of you may be asking, "If I am following everything I am being told to do, why am I becoming sicker, fatter and more depressed as the years pass by?" If you have asked yourself this question after being prescribed medication after medication and being told, "You just have to think positive and eat more fruits and vegetables!" as both Michelle and I were told, you are not alone. Is patient adherence and motivation the problem, or could it simply be the advice we are being given is not the right answer?

So enters the dilemma, as Michelle Hurn, RD LD, so poignantly asks in the opening of her book: "What would you do if your health was restored by doing the opposite of everything you were taught?" In the field of medicine, we adhere to guidelines that are put in place based on the best scientific evidence, to ensure our patients obtain the best health outcomes. In *The Dietitian's Dilemma*, Michelle explores one set of guidelines in particular: our food guidelines. Does the "one size fits all" food pyramid work for everyone? Or are there other options, such as low-carbohydrate and ketogenic diets that may mitigate our risk for metabolic illness, or even better, restore us to health? After years on a high-carbohydrate diet, intense running sessions, struggling with an eating disorder, in the throes of anxiety and depression to the point of suicidal ideation, Michelle knew she needed a change.

Chancing upon Ultra Runner Zach Bitter, she started a meat-based, low-carbohydrate diet, following a nutrition approach opposite to what she was taught in school and what she recommended to her patients. Within weeks, Michelle's severe muscle pain and anxiety disappeared. Eager to learn more, Michelle researched and soon found overwhelming data supporting the use of low-carbohydrate diets in weight loss, diabetes, as well as anecdotal evidence and case reports for improved mental health. In my experience, it is the natural inclination of most health care providers to want to share this information with patients who may benefit from this option. Unfortunately, Michelle's research was met with resistance from her peers and she was bound to practice within a set of guidelines that had not yet evolved with the current evidence she was researching. If you are wondering what this dilemma feels like for most healthcare providers, it is the equivalent of a hostage situation at all times.

As Michelle says in her insightful book, one of the most empowering things you can do is share through your journey. Guiding her reader in their own search for truth, Michelle opens the book sharing her deeply intimate, personal story. I cried reading it. Unfortunately, Michelle's journey is not unique, but her voice is amplified by the testimonies of others throughout the pages of this book. During my own journey, I wondered, "Why was I not given this information sooner and saved years of suffering?" The simple answer is, *You don't know what you don't know.* If you do not know literature supporting other dietary options exist, you will not know to search for it. This book, *The Dietitian's Dilemma,* pulls back the veil for readers to explore current nutrition research and ask questions. What this book is not, is an attack on modern medicine, medical professions or individual lifestyles. It is a book that invites us all to critically consider the nutrition options science has afforded us in our quest for optimal health. It is the book you wished you had when you started your journey.

The chapters that unfold take you on a riveting journey of the evidence and the role nutrition plays in diabetes, heart disease, mental health, eating disorders, sarcopenia and cholesterol. You will clearly see the dietitian's dilemma, as the literature does not mirror the patient's plate at home or in practice. You may ask yourself, "Where did our Dietary Guidelines come from? Surely they are rooted in robust scientific data?" The shocking truth, as Michelle reveals, is that the guidelines were the result of political power, corporate profit and opinions repetitively marketed to the general public, so much so that they eventually became disguised as ingrained, unrefuted facts.

The Dietitian's Dilemma provides an opportunity for both health care providers and patients to think critically about the way we view and treat metabolic illnesses. Sparking curiosity, Michelle challenges us to develop an approach that looks for the root cause of disease, implementing dietary and lifestyle intervention, versus the initial opting for a medical bandage. Michelle has paved the way for the beginning of an open dialogue and civil discourse regarding evidence-based nutrition options available to help our patients return to a life of health and purpose. She is also equally open to the fact that we still have a lot of work to do, and addresses questions that require further research and study. In her chapter, *Getting Started*, Michelle offers the pros and cons of what she considers the 3 tiers of low-carbohydrate nutrition, as well as safety measures that health care providers and patients should watch for in terms of medication, hormone and electrolyte management. Patient empowerment and provider education are themes that consistently run throughout *The Dietitian's Dilemma*. Michelle encourages the development of rewarding relationships between patients and healthcare providers.

What book would be complete without a happy ending for the reader and the author? Michelle's story, just like yours, does not end with this book. It is only beginning.

Nevada Gray, PharmD, R.N.

My Story

I stood in front of the mirror gazing back at my expression. I was cold; bitterly, painfully cold. I had grown accustomed to being cold, but the aching in my muscles was becoming too much to bear. I'll never forget how my eyes looked in the mirror. I've seen that glossy, hopeless look many times now, since that fateful day in March of 1995. *Who is this monster?* I thought. *I don't recognize this person at all.* My eyes were distant and cloudy, a sign that my body was losing the war within me. My spirit felt broken, but my body was still fighting to keep me alive. I slammed my fist into the mirror as tears ran down my face. *It doesn't matter anyway.* I had heard what the doctor said. My suffering would be over soon. I sat against the wall taking deep breaths as I attempted to mentally unravel the knot in my chest. *If there is a God, if a higher being truly exists, He won't let me suffer much longer*, I assured myself. I closed my eyes. *Breathe in, breathe out. It will be over soon.*

****

I grew up in Plano, Texas, right outside of Dallas. I am the youngest of four girls and from an early age, I was quite the tomboy. I loved sports, competition, and getting dirty. It was not unusual for me to come home with scraped knees or a black eye from playing full contact football with the older boys in my neighborhood. My next oldest sister, Kristen, is 14 months older than I am. Growing up, she and I were inseparable. We spent hours playing with stuffed animals and pretending to be Ninja Turtles. My second oldest sister, Heather, is four years older than me. As far back as I can remember, I admired Heather greatly. She has always been brilliant and driven. Today she is an accomplished business owner, surgeon, and parent. My oldest sister, Stephanie, invited me into her home during my later teens and early twenties. Her strength, kindness, and work ethic reinforced the importance of compassion and determination during a particularly difficult time in my early adulthood.

Growing up, I witnessed my mom experience oscillating bouts of mania followed by crippling depression. It was not unusual for my mom to go from working 12-hour shifts waiting tables or stocking shelves to cleaning our entire house compulsively. She would be in constant motion until she would collapse from exhaustion. Her severe anxiety refused to let her rest. In between these bouts of Energizer Bunny-type energy, and resulting exhaustion, I watched her grapple with an unseen enemy. At five feet four inches and barely 100 pounds, she was convinced she was "too fat."

Growing up, my older sisters and I had front row seats to her severe struggles with eating. From the time I was five years old, I watched my mom restrict her food to bite-sized portions and extremely low-calorie items, then proceed to give into hunger and binge on high-calorie treats, such as cookies or cake. This was followed by screaming, crying, throwing things, and berating herself for indulging in, "bad foods." Without realizing what she was doing, my mother was teaching that food had strong moral implications. If you ate "good" foods you were good. If you ate "bad" foods you were bad. In my developing mind, being fat equated to being unlovable. From very early on, I was being wired to have a dysfunctional relationship with food, weight, and coping mechanisms. Things got progressively worse as I got older.

My mother is college educated and had the relevant experience to become a teacher, yet her bipolar disorder, depression, and severe anxiety made it difficult for her to pursue teaching. She found refuge in working jobs with simple, repetitive tasks. Unfortunately, these jobs tended to be physically demanding, and they barely paid minimum wage. Despite her education and experience, she ended up working the graveyard shift, stocking shelves at Walmart or waiting tables at IHOP. Often, she appeared frightened, exhausted, and overwhelmed. I remember thinking many times as a young child that perhaps there would be less sadness and financial struggle within my family if I had never been born. I was told more than once that I was a "surprise child" and that, "we certainly didn't want another right after your sister was born." I learned it was best to keep quiet and pretend everything was going fine as much as possible. This was an exercise in inauthenticity that would take years to work through.

As I entered middle school, I started to struggle with my body as it began to change. Although I did well in school, I felt socially awkward. I did not feel like I fit in with the boys or the girls. I started playing competitive soccer, and I felt like I had finally found a niche. However, before I even knew what was happening, it all fell apart.

At that time, I was eating the "normal" Standard American Diet. I would have cereal for breakfast, pizza for lunch at school, and we usually sat down together as a family for dinner. When Mom began working nights stocking shelves at Walmart, she would often be asleep before my sisters and I woke up for breakfast and school. As my 6th grade year continued, we stopped having dinner as a family. With no adults around for any of my meals, I started eating more haphazardly.

On the soccer field, a well-meaning parent told me I looked "lean and mean." It was the first time in a long time I had received a compliment from a parental figure. I remember thinking that if I could exercise a bit more and eat a little less, perhaps I could get "leaner and meaner". I decided to start tracking calories and limit myself to a few small snacks a day. Within weeks I was outrunning everyone on the soccer field. I was fast and unstoppable. It was an incredible high. Finally, something in my life felt good. I was getting the attention and positive reinforcement I so desperately desired. I was on top of the world.

As you can imagine, it was short lived. As the weeks went on, I began to feel sore, weak, and exhausted. I could not focus in school. My straight A record fell to B's, and then C's. Sitting down hurt, and I started to get weird bruises on my back. A phenomenon that will likely be difficult to understand, unless you have experienced it, happened during this time. My body image became severely distorted. I looked in the mirror and was horrified at the morbidly obese person staring back at me. I could feel my ribs sticking out, but the reflection in the mirror did not line up with what I could tangibly feel. I weighed myself several times a day and tracked calories meticulously. I had notebooks filled with foods, calories, weight, and comments. My arbitrary goal became less than 200 calories a day. Diet Coke, gum, and coffee became my best friends. It was easy to skip breakfast and dinner since we didn't sit down to eat as a family; no one noticed. Skipping lunch at school was more challenging, but I developed a routine where I would walk around the entire school and then hide in the bathroom and read during lunch period.

As the bones in my face and hips began to visibly protrude, I became an easy target for jokes and physical punishment from other kids. I became good at withstanding and compartmentalizing the physical abuse. During one recess break, the leader of a group of bullies pushed me onto the concrete so hard that I cracked my elbow. I said nothing. I simply got up, went to the school nurse's office, and asked for some ice. When she asked what happened, I simply stated, "It was my fault. I fell." My limited self-esteem was slowly unraveling, and my brain was so malnourished that I was unable to see beyond my current circumstance. As the physical abuse and name-calling continued, my low self-esteem turned into self-hatred.

My only refuge during this time became the high of starvation. While everything around me felt like it was crumbling, restricting food made me feel strangely at peace and in control. My grades were abysmal, I had quit soccer, and I pushed my sisters and friends away. I was being physically and emotionally abused on a daily basis. I felt completely and hopelessly alone.

One day, I was walking to class when I started to feel dizzy. I had a strange feeling like I was going to throw up and suddenly everything went black. I woke up in a hospital where I was told my blood glucose level was 24. At the time I did not understand what that meant, but now I realize a blood sugar level that low can result in death. While I was lying in the hospital bed, I was questioned by a police officer. His face was serious, but his words were kind. He calmly asked if my parents were abusing me. I remember thinking this was a really odd question. "No, of course not! Why?" I asked. He went on to ask why my back was covered in bruises and why my elbow was swollen. He also asked if there was enough food in my house. This was not my parents; fault, and now they were being blamed! I remember feeling tremendous guilt and shame.

I began to dread going to school. My body was constantly tense from anxiety and obsessive, racing thoughts regarding food and weight. With less body fat than before, I was bruising easier. I went from feeling uncomfortably cold to *painfully cold*. My hair was falling out, and my muscles ached.

The anger, yelling, begging, pleading, and bargaining around food by my concerned family fell on deaf and profoundly ill ears. I was too far gone. I continued to starve myself until I was admitted to an inpatient eating disorder facility in Wickenburg, Arizona.

When I arrived at Remuda Ranch, I was just under 5 feet tall and I weighed just shy of 57.5 pounds. For those of you who use the metric system this is 150 cm and 26.1 kilograms. My body mass index was 11.7. Multiple tests revealed my heart was failing, my kidneys were shutting down, and all my electrolytes, including blood glucose, were dangerously low. I continued to have severe body dysmorphia, and I felt shame and disgust over the person I saw in the mirror.

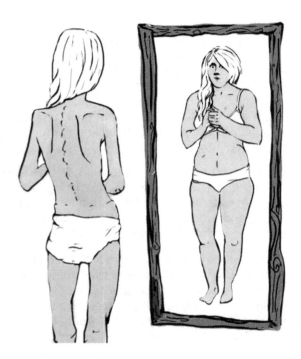

After the battery of tests and seemingly endless questions, the facility's doctor informed me that he needed to speak with my parents privately. Once they went behind closed doors, I snuck up to the door and pressed my ear against it, straining to hear the conversation. "Mr. and Mrs. Hurn, I am so sorry. This doesn't look good. It's rare we see someone so frail recover. If she does, it's likely she won't be able to do normal things again, like run or play. She may have permanent heart failure or kidney damage. She may never develop fully as a woman or grow beyond her current height." The room on the other side of the door was completely silent. I heard the doctor let out a sigh, and I will never forget the words he spoke next, "You need to be ready. There's a less than 10% chance that she will survive, and complete recovery is even more unlikely. I'm so, so sorry."

I wasn't actually there to get better. I was there to die. Perhaps I would die a bit more comfortably there than I would at home. Maybe my parents didn't want to be present when I actually passed away?

What I experienced next was one of the most difficult things I will ever choose to publicly admit or to put on paper.

At that very moment, I wasn't scared, angry, or upset. *I was overcome with relief.*

I wouldn't have to live like this much longer. My life and my suffering would soon come to an end! As I watched my parents drive away in their rental car, back to the airport, back to Texas, I remember feeling a surge of relief. I believed my existence was causing my parents tremendous sadness, and I was glad they would no longer feel anguish on my account.

Breathe in. Breathe out. It will be over soon.

The medical staff at Remuda Ranch saved my life. Throughout this book, I am critical of the current nutrition guidelines for my profession and of many Registered Dietitians. I will point to examples of how our health care system often uses medication as a band aid for chronic conditions. I discuss how most medications not only fail to address the root causes of disease, but they often have side effects that can lead to other, often more devastating diseases. For a chronic illness, trusting a well-meaning but poorly informed medical professional may keep you in the hospital or land you in the morgue.

The day after my parents dropped me off at Remuda Ranch, I was immediately put on a 24-hour tube feeding system and required to eat three mandatory meals per day. Even today, almost 25 years later, standard tube feeding formulas still contain the same basic ingredients that I was fed during my hospitalization.

> Standard Tube Feeding Ingredient list: Water, corn maltodextrin, corn syrup solids, sodium caseinate, canola oil, corn oil, short-chain fructooligosaccharides, soy protein isolate, medium chain triglycerides, calcium caseinate, oat fiber. Less than 0.5% of soy fiber, vitamin and mineral blend.

As the weeks went on, my calories and carbohydrates increased. I was tube fed over 400 grams of processed carbohydrates, and I was prescribed seven different medications to treat anxiety, depression, headaches, nausea, and diarrhea.

My inpatient stay at Remuda Ranch is where I encountered my first dietitian. She was a strange lady with a whispery, mouse-like voice and a terrible haircut. I found her lack of macronutrient memorization and explanation of the food exchange system to be inadequate and ill-informed. After our second meeting I thought she should know that her incompetence was irritating.

"Someday I'm going to be dietitian and I'll be a hell-a lot better that you," I informed her. To her credit, she laughed at my insult. She smiled and simply responded, "Sounds good, but you're going to have to get better first. I hope you do."

Prior to the summer of my 14th birthday, I had a physical examination with my family doctor. I was about 70 pounds and still terribly underweight. I told the doctor it was my goal to play sports again. I remember he laughed at me, commenting, "I'm not signing off on you running around! You could have a heart attack." He went on to tell my parents that my heart rate was still too low, and I was still dangerously underweight.

After the appointment, I was confined to the house for the entire summer. Without the freedom to come and go, I started to spend more time at home with my sister Kristen. As you may recall, she is a mere 14 months older than I am, and we had been best friends prior to my eating disorder. At that time, I was still holding onto many eating disordered tendencies, such as keeping a list of foods which I considered "forbidden." I was known to avoid high-fat foods such as pizza like the plague. One hot summer day, Kristen came home from her job at a local pizza joint with a few friends and a large pepperoni pizza. She and her friends were all digging in as I walked into the kitchen and asked, out of nowhere, if I could have a slice. I do not exaggerate when I say the room went dead silent.

From then on, that summer, I made it my number one goal to challenge my food fears. Kristen and I biked to our local fast-food joints, and I would eat a burgers and fries. The leftover pizza Kristen brought home became a nightly, post-dinner treat. Kristen and I biked to our local health food store, and she bought me a high calorie, protein drink mix. Even mixed with ice cream, it tasted terrible, but I drank it every day. I slowly started to put on some muscle and gain back the weight I had lost over the last few years. Before my freshman year of high school, at age of 14, I went to my family doctor's office for another physical. "I want to play sports," I had told my parents. I waited patiently in the doctor's office, knowing this time the end result would be a little different, and I was given the go-ahead.

With renewed vigor, I tried out for the basketball team my freshman year of high school. I was short, uncoordinated, and not particularly good at shooting hoops, so I was cut. The basketball coach told me she could help me enroll in P.E. I did not want to take P.E.! "What if I try out for soccer or softball?" I pleaded. Then, the basketball coach said something that would change my life: "Why don't you sign up for the running thing? You could get your energy out and stop bothering me." I had no idea what "the running thing" was, but I was intrigued.

The first day of cross-country practice, I showed up in cotton shorts and basketball shoes. Despite the searing mid-August Texas heat, I immediately fell in love with running. I loved to explore, compete, and push myself. There was something peaceful about jogging down the quiet streets early in the morning. I liked how my body felt after running. I felt tired yet accomplished. Running with a team gave me comradery, confidence, and something positive to put my energy into. I had a new reason to feed and fuel my body, and I liked seeing my body grow stronger. I was part of a team, and I loved it.

I discovered I had a knack for running long distances. I was not particularly fast, but I could run for a long time without tiring. My very first race was a 5-mile road race. My legs hurt, my lungs hurt, and I really wanted to quit, but I persisted. It was terrible and wonderful at the same time. After crossing the finish line, I felt something I had not felt for a while. Pride.

As time went on, life seemed to be going great. I started working with a club coach, and I was running faster than ever. I also took a job at a local smoothie place, and started learning about the relationship between amino acids and muscle growth. I was getting straight A's in school, and at the age of 15, I won the 3,200m at the Texas state track meet.

My club coach told me that I could get a scholarship if I performed well my junior and senior years. Growing up without a lot of money, a scholarship seemed like an ideal solution to constant financial worry. I had put a tremendous amount of work into rebuilding my body, and now I was the fastest high schooler in Texas. As a 15-year-old, I was running twice a day Monday through Thursday and once a day Friday through Sunday. I worked at the smoothie place Fridays after school and during the day on Saturdays and Sundays. I was eating a lot of protein and total calories. I wasn't restricting food, and I was sleeping well. What could possibly go wrong?

My club coach pushed me hard during the summer before my junior year. He kept asking me if I "really wanted," that scholarship. While friends were eating ice cream and hanging out at the pool, I was running around the track in 100-degree heat. He reminded me that "leanness equaled quickness". At the time I was around 10% body fat, but I began to believe I could be faster if I was leaner. While doing some nutrition research, I heard that being a vegetarian could help improve running performance and help people "lean out." I liked protein, and at the time I was eating meat twice a day, and supplementing with whey protein powder.

I started journaling about breaking the two mile and mile state records. I became laser focused. I decided I would do whatever was necessary to secure my scholarship. I began to eat a steady diet of fruit, salads, bagels and oatmeal. I bought some soy protein powder that tasted terrible, but I dutifully chugged it down twice a day. If my family was having meat or any food that involved meat, I would just eat around it. I felt proud of myself thinking I was getting "tons of vitamins and minerals" from my high vegetable diet.

From the outside, things seemed really good. I ended up losing almost 10 pounds and I did, indeed, become faster. I ended up being 4th in the Junior Nationals competition and was ranked as one of the fastest women in the US for my age. On the inside, however, I started to have severe anxiety again. I began to have shin splints and my right hamstring became so chronically painful that I had to ice it throughout the day. Sleep no longer came easily. I'd often lay in bed until 1 or 2 am, only to finally fall asleep and wake up to a blaring alarm at 5:00am. I became an unpleasant person to be around, and my grades started to suffer.

During this time, not one person suggested that my diet or weight loss could be part of the problem.

I continued to eat a steady diet of plain bread, raw fruits, raw vegetables and soy protein powder.

During my junior year, my high school coach pulled me into her office to confront me about my weight loss. I was so incredibly stubborn and not particularly kind during those years. I had such little control over so many aspects of my life that I viewed anyone questioning my eating habits or running as ignorant or jealous of what it took to be successful. At this point, I had stopped having my period for over a year, but I had not told anyone. I had read an article that hard endurance training could cause women to miss periods. At that age, I did not understand how important ovulating and hormonal regulation was for bone health. I assured my coach that I was "just fine" and she would be better served focusing on other athletes on the team.

A week later, a body composition test provided me with tangible results that things were not only *not* "just fine," but I was headed down a dangerous path.

Just like when I was 12, I had begun to get bruises on my back and tailbone from sitting in class. I was constantly hungry, bloated, and had blood in my stool. *Was this what it took to be an elite athlete?*

My body fat was 5.7%, which was deemed "dangerously low; seek medical advice" on a print-out I had received with my results. I shared this print-out with my current club coach and asked him, point blank, if such a low body fat percentage was okay. He dismissed my concerns and praised me for my dedication. He confirmed it wouldn't be long before I was breaking college records. "Keep pushing hard, and you'll be competing on a national level in no time."

Everything changed during my senior year of high school. After a particularly long morning run, I ended up sprinting to my next class to avoid being late. As I stepped off a curb mid-sprint, I felt a sharp, stabbing pain in my hip. As I attempted to jog it off, it felt like the pain was radiating down my leg. While I was familiar with shin splints, hamstring strains, and all kinds of muscle soreness, this was a sensation that intuitively told me I needed to stop.

When I tried to run the next day, I felt the same unbearable pain in that same hip. It felt like someone was stabbing me, and it was sending shock waves down my leg.

An X-ray revealed I had a clear break through the pubis ramus bone. The doctor told me, "It's significant. We need to set you up with a bone density scan." I was told that this type of break wasn't normal for someone my age, and I would be on crutches for at least 12 weeks.

I felt like someone had just punched me in the chest! *Broken hip? Doesn't that happen to frail, 80-year-old grandmas? What about my scholarship?* **Who am I** *without running?*

The results of the bone density test were worse than I had anticipated. I had osteopenia in my hips an osteoporosis in my spine. To say I felt devastated and completely lost would be a gross understatement; I had no idea what to do next.

Not surprisingly, all running scholarship offers were off the table. College athletics is a business, and no coach in his or her right mind would take a chance on a teenager with osteoporosis.

In desperation, I called a local club coach named Terry and asked if he could help me. We set up a meeting where he kindly but firmly laid some ground rules. Eating enough calories and having meat daily was non-negotiable. I was also to "stop being so serious," in his words. He was concerned that I was basing my entire identity on how fast I could run and getting a scholarship. He was not wrong. It felt like someone was finally giving me permission to *chill the fuck out*. It gave me an odd sense of relief.

I ended up getting a partial academic scholarship to the University of Arkansas. I walked on to the cross-country team, and I had incredible time as a freshman.

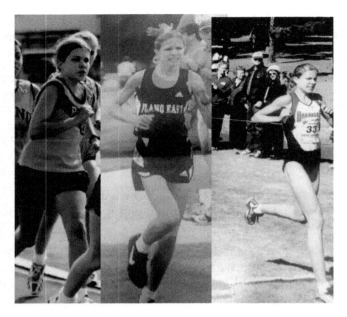

From left to right: freshman in high school, junior in highschool, freshman in college

A week before the cross-country national race, I felt a strange shift and sharp pain in the back of my hip. It didn't feel like the pain I had experienced when I fractured my hip in high school, but it was constant. I was looked at by the trainer and ended up seeing the team doctor. Concerned for a possible stress fracture, my coach had me get an X-ray. Everything checked out fine. The pain continued, so I ended up getting an MRI with contrast, which showed a severe stress fracture in my left iliac crest. The doctor told me he had been practicing for 38 years and this was only the second iliac crest fracture he had ever seen; the first one was an 80-year-old woman who had been T-boned in a bad car accident. This diagnosis would effectively be the end of my running career at the University of Arkansas.

Over the next few years, I ran minimally, and focused on finishing my degree. I was accepted to the Dietetic Internship program at Oregon Health & Science University, which is a prominent teaching hospital in Portland, Oregon. This seemed like the perfect place to springboard me into a career as a dietitian.

Before the internship started, I started running more frequently. I quickly found that I had missed the wonderful source of stress relief that running provided.

In August of 2007, I met a woman named Corene. She was cute, cocky, confident, and really sweet. At the end of our third date, we mutually decided we wouldn't continue to date. However, we ended up in the same group of friends, and as the years went on, we found ourselves falling in love. Seven years later, I proposed to Corene, and we were married shortly afterwards. She's the most incredible person I know and I'm incredibly lucky.

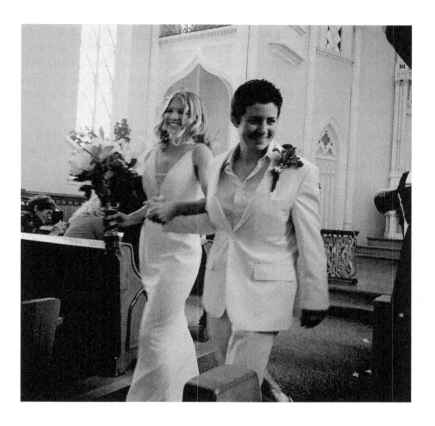

As a young dietitian, I was quite sure that the key to health was blood sugar stability. I was taught that if your blood sugar is too high or too low, you can become very ill. There was data to support that a balance of high-quality protein, from either animals or plants, with lots of vegetables for fiber, and low glycemic carbohydrates, could potentially lead to "normal" blood sugar levels. At this point, I believed carbohydrates and fiber were necessary components for health. Despite my beliefs, I saw a disconnect between the information I had been taught and the health of my current patients. Many patients were dutifully eating "healthy" whole grains, fruit, vegetables, and lean protein, yet they continued to be sick, diabetic, and obese.

When I questioned my colleagues if carbohydrates were truly necessary for health, I was met with incredible resistance from fellow dietitians and other health professionals. I was still new to practicing as a dietitian, so I continued to encourage foods that aligned with the status quo.

I took a job working as an acute dietitian. Working in acute care, I would see patients who were admitted to the hospital with immediate, pressing issues, such as infections. These issues were often caused by poor management of chronic diseases such as diabetes, heart disease, or kidney failure. I would imagine that when most people hear the word "dietitian" they picture an individual sitting down with patients and going over meal plans. Perhaps this individual reviews the patient's current way of eating, answers questions about carbohydrates, fat, and protein, and uses motivational interviewing to discuss how the patient can overcome barriers to change.

As an acute care dietitian, your only goal is to keep the patient alive. That's it. You're only allotted the time and resources to address a single point, which is, "Is the patient getting enough protein and calories?"

This is the major concern of the acute care dietitian. The source of calories the patient is eating is mostly irrelevant. If we can get a patient to consume a highly processed, fruit-flavored gelatin with 44 grams of sugar and a small amount added protein, this is considered "great." A high-sugar, boxed juice drink with added vitamins and soy protein is considered an "excellent" supplement. We are told that the patient will have to see an outpatient dietitian should they want to address their chronic nutrition issues. Our only goal as acute care dietitians is to have people eat or drink calories and protein.

I remember early in my career going into each patient's room with the goal to discuss dietary strategies, but I was quickly alerted that we are, "only interested in the immediate problem." If a patient has recently lost weight or has a poor appetite, we will speak with that patient. We spend 5 minutes (tops) discussing their appetite, encouraging them to eat pretty much anything they want because the ultimate goal is protein and calories. The nutritional quality of the food they are eating is considered to be a low priority in these cases.

While I do occasionally provide nutritional education, the nutrition advice I'm required to present is the Academy of Nutrition Guidelines. Often, these carbohydrate-heavy guidelines are a cause of the patient becoming overweight and ill in the first place. I felt frustrated when I was instructed to discuss carbohydrate counting with my diabetic patients. Why were we advocating that diabetics eat 75-90 grams of carbohydrates at each meal (which will substantially raise blood sugar) and then having them take medications to then lower their blood sugar? Why not remove carbohydrates from their diets? This could eliminate the need for medication and restore their blood sugar levels to normal.

Carbohydrates, while not essential for the human body, are the base of the nutrition pyramid (nutrition guidelines), and prescribing them to all patients,

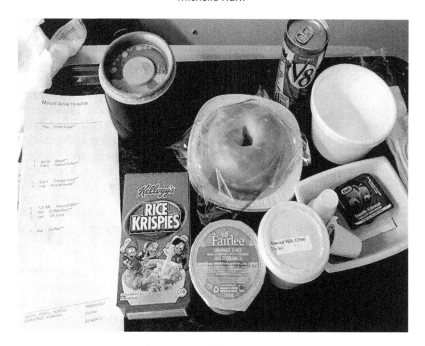

Actual Patient Breakfast in the Hospital

regardless of disease state, was non-negotiable. At this time, discussing a low-carbohydrate diet with a patient was considered "dangerous and unethical."

I had spent my entire life and education wanting to help people with nutrition, and now I found myself writing orders for high calorie, high fructose corn syrup-laden, boxed meal-replacement drinks TID (three times a day) with meals. Every patient a dietitian sees requires at least thirty minutes of extensive chart notes to fulfill documentation requirements. I became disheartened with the profound disconnect between what information could help people and what information I was required to teach. I also had a huge patient load, and very little time to actually talk to my patients. I brought up these concerns to my first Clinical Director. Her words summed up our flawed health care system: "The patient will have to get outpatient help on their own time." It wasn't my job to help anyone; I just needed to keep checking boxes.

I continued to do everything I could to ensure my sanity while working in the hospital setting. I even took a short hiatus to sell real estate and help a friend work in a local café. In 2017, I trained with my close friend who is an Elite Marathon Runner, and I ran the fastest marathon of my life. I clocked a 2.54.32 at the California International Marathon. This time was less than 10 minutes away from qualifying for the Olympic trials. I was confident I was on the right track, but slowly, once again, things began to unravel.

At the age of 36, my body stopped recovering well from workouts. I started doubling my iron supplementation, eating more calories, and prioritizing sleep. My easy runs were going okay, but anytime I ran over two hours or did a track workout, I would be painfully sore for several days. I decided to double down on the amount of carbohydrates I was eating. I felt exhausted, bloated, and dizzy stuffing myself with bread and bananas, but I felt marginally better on my long runs and workouts. I struggled falling asleep, and I often woke up two to three times a night. Some nights it was like being in college again where I would wake up at 1 or 2AM and be unable to fall back asleep.

I reached out to two different sports dietitians during this time to see if they had any feedback regarding the symptoms I was experiencing. I asked each of these dietitians point-blank if they thought the amount of carbohydrates I was eating could be contributing to my fatigue, bloating or anxiety. *Both dismissed the idea.* They encouraged me to continue a high-carbohydrate diet because, "the body needs carbohydrates for energy." One of these dietitians told me I should consider having more frequent snacks. I was eating 5-6 times a day at that point. Her advice was to increase the meal and snack frequency to 7-8 times a day.

Like many periods throughout my adolescence and adulthood, my anxiety flared up again. I began to feel hopeless, and for the first time in several years I started to feel suicidal. I agreed to see my family practice doctor.

She ran a simple blood test which showed I was deficient in magnesium. "Eat more spinach," she said, and then she recommended I increase my dosage of antidepressants. I left her office feeling angry and even more frustrated than before. Intuitively, I knew a few handfuls of spinach and doubling up on Lexapro was not the answer to what was becoming debilitating anxiety. At least I had my running as a coping mechanism.

Then, what seemed like overnight, my running fell off a cliff.

I went out to run a routine eight-mile easy run. Two miles into the run, I broke out in a cold sweat and felt like I might throw up right there on the spot. I had certainly experienced overheating or fatigue during longer, hot weather efforts, but this was a short run on a cool day. I stopped immediately and walked home. When I arrived home, my stomach felt like it was doing backflips. The nausea was so severe I had to sit down on the floor for several minutes.

At the time, I didn't understand what was happening. Now, I can see that my body was overresponding to the amount of carbohydrates I was eating. I had been eating so many carbohydrates for so long, that my pancreas was actually producing too much insulin in an attempt to shuttle the glucose out of my blood stream and into my cells. *Years of excessive carbohydrate intake, high intensity exercise, and poor stress management had finally caught up with me.*

My attempts to run over the next two weeks proved futile. My muscles ached, and I felt like I was trudging through quicksand. I started to have really awful back and leg pain. The final straw came about a week later. I had had a particularly difficult day at work, and I came home feeling frustrated and sad. I ended up falling asleep early, but I woke up to searing pain at 2AM. My leg muscles felt like they were on fire.

I decided I would soak in an ice bath. So around 2:30AM I drove to our local gas station to get three 10-pound bags of ice. As quietly as possible, I placed them in the bathtub, and filled the remainder of the tub with cold water. It was 3AM and there I was, sitting in an ice-cold bath, tears streaming down my face. I remember thinking, "What am I doing with my life?" My wife came in and sat next to the bathtub. She looked at me and very calmly stated, "Maybe it's time to think about doing something differently." It was past that time. I decided at that moment my running days were done.

I began to make peace with my new fate. I simply was too old to continue to compete in long distance running. Now that I was no longer competing, I decided I could back off on the carbohydrates. I had heard that a ketogenic diet could help inflammation, but I was worried my energy would be low on a carbohydrate restricted diet.

I decided that since my running days were over, I'd go low-carb or no-carb for a few weeks to see if it could help my muscle inflammation and pain. I continued to do research on the ketogenic diet and while doing so I came across an athlete named Zach Bitter. He is an Ultra-endurance runner, eating a high-meat, high-fat, relatively low carbohydrate diet. He isn't just an average runner. He currently holds the world record for the fastest ever 100-mile run. For his world record, he ran the equivalent of four marathons back-to-back at a pace that would have qualified for the Boston Marathon if he had run *any* of them individually. *How in the world was he thriving and breaking records on a low-carbohydrate diet?*

As I continued to research a low-carbohydrate diet, I came across a former orthopedic surgeon named Shawn Baker. Dr. Baker was literally *only* eating meat and fat. He didn't consume any carbohydrates or plants in his diet, and he broke records in rowing. He wrote an entire book on what he called "The Carnivore Diet." I could get behind a low-carbohydrate diet and I liked the idea of more fat. But, no fruits or vegetables, ever? *Only* meat and fat?

I decided I would send Zach Bitter an email asking for more information on his running and way of eating. If his diet could keep inflammation low enough that he could dominate long distance running, could it also reverse diseases of chronic inflammation for my patients? Could it help my now chronic, low-grade muscle pain?

Zach emailed me back right away. He explained that he used carbohydrates as, "rocket fuel" only. He reserved them for high intensity training and racing, and he kept his carbohydrate intake relatively low during recovery days and low intensity exercise. This man was running over 100 miles a week and eating less than 25% of the amount of carbohydrates my psychiatric and hospital patients were eating on a *daily basis.* While he was thriving, they continued to get sicker. Could this purely be a coincidence?

Since I was already interested in a low-carbohydrate way of eating and because I love meat, I thought why not give a meat-only diet a try? I thought I would do it for a few weeks, just to see if the extra protein might help my muscles heal.

To say my wife was initially not on board with this way of eating would be a *huge understatement.* We fought bitterly about this. Corene's resistance was understandable as she had watched me struggle with anxiety around food for years. She had witnessed me create various meal plans, most of which were disordered ways to limit total calories and food volume. She viewed an all-meat diet, even if it was for a short period of time, to be a highly restrictive, eating disordered regimen.

"This will only set you back in your recovery," she declared angrily. "Let me get this straight, you literally want to eat *just* meat and fat? Why can't you just have *some* carbohydrates? Just... less?" She was frustrated, and I hated seeing her upset.

"Just for now," I said. "I just have to see if this can help me stop hurting."

But Corene was having none of it. She cried, which made me feel terrible. After a few more days of arguing, she asked me to come sit and talk. "You're an adult, you can do whatever you want. I'll be here when you quit, because this won't last long," she confidently informed me.

As the days went on, I slowly started to feel less physical pain. I also noticed I was feeling a sense of calm, which was refreshing. When I opened up to my dietitian colleagues about this way of eating, I was immediately pegged as a weirdo. "How will you get enough vitamins and minerals?" they demanded. Aren't you concerned that your heart will explode with all that fat? Wouldn't all that meat cause widespread systemic inflammation? Will you be able to poop without fiber?" My coworkers seemed to rally around the fact that this diet might help me with an endurance event. "So surely after this event you'll stop eating all this meat, right? *You wouldn't eat like this forever, would you?"*

Heading into the third week of eating a mostly meat and fat-based diet, my wife asked if we could sit down and chat again. Her words were telling, "I'm not sure I like this way of eating," she began, "but this is the *best your anxiety has been in the eleven year I've known you.*"

It was true. I was feeling happy and calm again. I could eat a high-meat, high-fat breakfast and be completely satiated for 6-8 hours. It felt like a miracle! By the end of the fourth week, my muscles stopped hurting completely. I wasn't hungry or "hangry". I ate fatty cuts of beef with butter and two cups of coffee with heavy cream daily. We would occasionally have some chicken, pork, or salmon, but most of the time we opted for beef with extra tallow or butter. It was complete opposite of everything I had ever been taught about nutrition. Was this way of eating really the answer to my health concerns and further, could this help others?

A few weeks more went by and my wife and I started digging into the research on low-carbohydrate, animal-based diets. I was devouring every bit of information I could find on this way of eating and so was she.

At some point, she told me I was annoying her because I had too much energy. She made a comment that I should, "Go for a run." I hadn't really run in weeks, and I was scared. I had given up on being a "runner" and I didn't want to experience the debilitating muscle pain I had been living with just a few months ago.

"Okay, you know what?' I told her, "I'm just going to run a mile or two. It might be fun. You can't run long without carbs anyway." I put my hat on backwards, laced up my shoes, and left the house. I was planning to jog around the block a few times but ended up running eight miles without any issues.

I just ran 8 miles on a minimal-carbohydrate, high-meat, high-fat diet!

The wheels started spinning in my head. What was this? What was going on?

Then I got a crazy idea.

I decided to start an Instagram account dedicated to my running journey and healing my anxiety and muscle pain with a low-carbohydrate, animal-based diet. What would I call it? I decided on @RunEatMeatRepeat. The new story of my life. I was hopeful that I could rally a few hundred followers and spread information and advocacy for a diet that directly aligned with human physiology. In February of 2020, I was fortunate to be interviewed by an incredible woman, Caitlin Weeks, one of the prominent figures in the low-carbohydrate and ketogenic community. Her YouTube interview with me received over 12,000 views. My wife suggested I start my own YouTube channel, and after a lot of resistance, I decided to go for it. I started the "The Dietitian's Dilemma" channel, where I interview individuals who have completely changed their physical and mental health by incorporating a ketogenic, animal based, low-carb diet. One common theme that was impossible to ignore was that *every single person I interviewed stated,* "I wish I had known about this way of eating sooner." As you read through this book, please remember, it will challenge the current nutritional way of thinking. Considering that 70% of the population is overweight or obese, and 88% have some type of metabolic issue due in part overconsumption of highly processed carbohydrates and sugar, I'd say this challenge is long overdue.

In less than six months, I went from having chronic anxiety, searing muscle pain, and not being able to run for twenty minutes, to feeling joyful and confident, and having zero lingering muscle pain. Moreover, I've covered up to 30 miles at a time during my training runs. At the age of 37, my physical and mental health are the best they've ever been. I consistently sleep through the night, and I wake up feeling rested and excited to start my day. I'm a better partner to my wife, friend, runner, and I believe I'm a much better dietitian (although the hospital system might disagree).

My body is nourished, and my mind feels calm and able to handle stress. I'm rarely sick, and my general view in life is hopeful and optimistic. The chains of anxiety, worry, and obsession over food have been broken. I feel *free*.

It is my sincerest hope that you will find helpful information, guidance, and inspiration in this book. When I first heard about a lower carbohydrate, high-protein, high-fat way of eating, I genuinely thought it was crazy. What I have come to realize, however, is that our current nutritional guidelines are what's crazy. It's crazy to keep eating in a way that causes chronic illness, anxiety, depression, and obesity. Our current nutrition guidelines will keep you alive, but it may not be a life worth living. I encourage you to take the time to read this book in its entirety before you get started. I believe it's important that you understand the foundation of nutrition as it related to human physiology as well as the nuances.

How I fuel my body starts with the foundation I present in this book, but it is an evolving process. Depending on your current health and overall goals, your eating will likely start with a foundation, but the specifics will move and change as your goals change, and your life situation and health improves. Remember, this is *your* life and *your* journey. May it be one filled with the courage to change, to overcome, and to become the absolute best version of *you*.

Chapter 1

Diabetes: A Better Option Than Counting Carbs

"The inability of current (dietary) recommendations to control the epidemic of diabetes, the specific failure of the prevailing low-fat diets to improve obesity, cardiovascular risk, or general health and the persistent reports of some serious side effects of commonly prescribed diabetic medications, in combination with the continued success of the low-carbohydrate diets in the treatment of diabetes and metabolic syndrome without significant effects, point to the need for a reappraisal of dietary guidelines." (1)

There are two main types of diabetes, type 1 and type 2. Type 1 diabetes tends to occur in youth or early adolescence. Type 1 occurs when the body's system for fighting infection goes awry and attacks and destroys the insulin-producing beta cells of the pancreas. In a person with type 1 diabetes, the pancreas no longer produces insulin, and the individual must administer insulin into their body every time they eat carbohydrates. My nephew was diagnosed with type 1 diabetes at the age of 4. He had to get used to being stuck with needles 3-6 times a day when he consumed carbohydrate rich foods. While we are seeing the prevalence of type 1 diabetes increase, it is important to note that 90-95% of diabetic cases are type 2. (2)

Type 2 Diabetes used to be called "Adult-Onset Diabetes" since it was rarely seen in children. Now, with the exponential increase in processed carbohydrates, type 2 diabetes has increased 4.8% per year between 2002 and 2012. (3) The fastest growing demographic of obese humans are children ages 2-5. (2) The youngest individual I have seen personally in the hospital setting with type 2 diabetes just celebrated his 8th birthday. He was 4 feet 2 inches (127 cm) and 212 pounds (96.4 kg).

Type 2 diabetes is no joke. The list of complications that arise from this preventable and often reversible disease are staggering. Blindness, amputations, stroke, dementia, and neuropathy are just a few of the consequences of this disease. The annual global cost of diabetes is projected to be more than 800 billion U.S. dollars. At the rate we are going, it is estimated that 500 million people worldwide will have diabetes by 2030. I have been at the bedside of patients ravaged by infections after a diabetic amputation. I remember holding the hand of an elderly patient who had unmanaged type 2 diabetes. She was having a pain crisis from a large, infected wound that was not healing well due to high blood sugar. The wound was so deep it went all the way to the bone.

When it comes to diabetic related amputations, studies show that the mortality rate after a diabetic amputation is higher than most malignancies.

This means that you have a higher chance of dying after a diabetic amputation than many cancerous tumors. (4)

Diabetes is the

7th

leading cause of **death**
in the U.S.

As I am writing this, the standard nutrition approach for the treatment and prevention of diabetes is literally the definition of insanity:

Doing the same thing over and over again and expecting different results.

Our current approach is not only ineffective, but also expensive and can potentially cause the patient unnecessary harm. The amount of inflammation, subcutaneous and visceral fat storage, and long-term nerve damage caused by high blood sugar, also called hyperglycemia, is well understood by the medical community, but often poorly explained (if explained at all) to the patient. I believe a complete nutritional overhaul to lower fasting blood sugar levels and decrease inflammation should be the *first line of defense* in the treatment of diabetes. Often, the patient will agree to prescription metformin or an insulin regimen without questioning the side effects or long-term consequences.

As a clinical dietitian working in an acute care setting, I have witnessed the tears and heartbreak experienced by family members of a diabetic who would be wheelchair bound and tube fed for the remainder of their days due to a stroke. I had a patient who became septic, which means he had an infection in the blood stream, because he stepped on a piece of glass. He had no feeling in his feet due to diabetic neuropathy, so he did not come to the hospital for five days! By that time, the glass was impaled into his foot and it caused a massive, whole body, systemic infection. I have seen rotting teeth, muscle wasting, blindness, and severe nerve damage in diabetic patients as young as their early 40's.

Perhaps more disheartening is that the Academy of Nutrition frames diabetes as a "complicated problem." A recent article on their website stated, "Learning to manage diabetes is complicated so you may need four to five visits across three to six months. Also, yearly follow-ups are recommended." (5)

Does managing and reversing diabetes need to be complicated? It will become complicated if we ask patients to count, measure, and track everything they eat. It is common practice to give patients a long list of carbohydrate containing foods to consume in "consistent doses" alongside one or more medications. Then, the patient will be told to exercise moderately and consume sugar "in moderation." Even if the patient dutifully follows this regimen, including meticulously counting carbohydrates, taking medications as prescribed, and completing some type of daily exercise, they will likely continue to experience frequent bouts of high or low blood sugars. With this current standard of practice, it seems we are setting the patient up to fail.

Often, patients with type 2 diabetes are advised to keep high sugar-containing foods such as glucose tablets or apple juice close by. They are to take these foods immediately if they find that their blood sugar drops too low. A potential issue with this is that when a person's blood sugar becomes so low that they need a fast-acting carbohydrate like apple juice or a pure glucose tablet, you guarantee a stress response from the body.

Anytime we have this type of stress response, you are going to experience inflammation. Another issue with low blood sugar is that most patients do not know their blood sugar is low until it is *dangerously low* or they experience *severe hypoglycemia*. Severe hypoglycemia can cause a person to be dizzy, nauseated, or even have a seizure and become unconscious. Because of the severity of very low blood sugar, many health care professionals prefer to keep blood sugar on the higher side which can cause its own long-term complications.

Most patients I have seen express frustration over their attempts to their manage diabetes with eating low-fat foods including fruits and vegetables, engaging in exercising, and admittedly, succumbing to having sweets due to hunger and frustration. Often, they end up deciding to wave the proverbial white flag when it comes to managing diabetes. It is often easier just to continue eating the foods they are used to eating and take whatever medications are deemed necessary. Over my many years working with a diverse group of patients, I have discovered that many patients have no idea that carbohydrates, in any form, can potentially have a detrimental effect on the body.

I have had diabetics tell me they "eat healthy" and "limit carbohydrates." As we review what foods they eat on a daily basis, I discover that they eat fruit, rice, yogurt, and oatmeal. All of these foods are loaded with carbohydrates that eventually break down into sugar. To be clear, I am not blaming the patient. I believe our system and my profession have done a disservice in failing to provide a science-based explanation of what to eat to reverse diabetes and restore health. I am here to provide information, present options, and remind you that the human body has a tremendous capacity to heal if we provide it with the right foods.

Note that every time a diabetic has carbohydrates in meals and snacks this causes a surge in blood sugar similar to the table below:

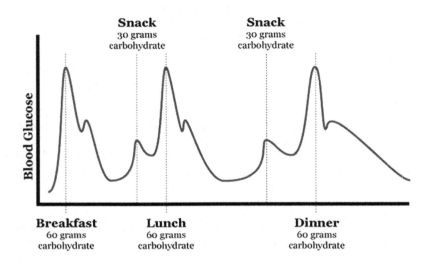

The good news is that there is a *much easier, incredibly effective* way to manage and potentially reverse diabetes. The better news is that, ultimately, it is possible to manage and reverse diabetes without having to track the carbohydrates you consume. Treating, and often reversing, diabetes is not easy because it requires a drastic change in the foods you eat and the foods you no longer eat. Change puts us outside of our comfort zones, which can feel scary and overwhelming. Over time, the changes that seemed overwhelming and daunting become routine. On the other side of fear, you might discover a quality of life that you did not even know was possible.

A theme you will notice throughout this book, and one I preach and practice in my profession, is a quote from the book *Strong Medicine*, by Blake F. Donaldson, "Really Important things have the strength of simplicity." (6) Treatment for individuals with type 2 diabetes has become unnecessarily complex, and I will present a more simple, straightforward approach.

I am certainly not the only medical professional who is fed up with the way we approach diabetes. Katherine Morrison, who published an article in the British Journal of General Practice writes, "It is time to stop feeding patients a diet of junk science and start feeling them food that makes them well instead of sick." (7) In other words, as Hippocrates put it, *Let food be thy medicine.*

Currently, the Academy of Nutrition recommends that diabetics be treated with a "consistent carbohydrate diet." This means we make sure patients have either 60 grams, 75 grams, or 90 grams of carbohydrates at each meal and 15-30 grams of carbohydrates as snacks. Following a consistent carbohydrate diet can add up to an individual consuming over 300 grams of carbohydrates a day. This is a very high amount of carbohydrates for someone who is unable to appropriately metabolize them to begin with. For reference, 300 grams of carbohydrates a day is the equivalent of a having two large pancakes with two tablespoons of maple syrup and an 8-ounce glass of orange juice for breakfast, 1 cup of pasta, two pieces of garlic bread, and a large banana for lunch, a granola bar for a snack, and a large sweet potato, a side of carrots, and a cookie with dinner.

What happens after a type 2 diabetic patient eats a set amount of carbohydrates at a meal or snack? The patient, a nurse, or a caregiver will inject an amount of insulin relative to the amount of carbohydrates the patient has eaten. How many units of insulin a diabetic needs to have injected into their body depends on how insulin-resistant their cells have become. Some patients need a significant amount of insulin to bring their blood sugar back to the normal range. It is important to note that this *is not an exact science*. It is not unusual for someone to receive an insulin injection and continue to have excessively high blood sugar. High blood sugar overtime is the number one cause of non-traumatic amputations. In fact, every day, 230 Americans will suffer a lower limb amputation due to complications from diabetes. (8) High blood sugar over time causes a slew of other medical complications including blindness, loss of feeling in the feet and limbs, and it can lead to heart or kidney failure. (9,10)

Some individuals with type 2 diabetes experience excessively low blood sugar after being injected with insulin. In this case, the person is given a fast-acting carbohydrate, like apple juice, to bring their blood sugar back up. Our current system has patients, nurses, and caregivers chasing blood sugar up and down, day in and day out, instead of putting a regimen in place that would permanently address and correct the root cause of diabetes.

In the 1960s, taking 50 units of insulin was considered "an excessive amount." Today, it is not unusual for someone to take 100-150 units of insulin a day. As shown in the chart below, the cost of insulin has skyrocketed over the last decade. Someone receiving 150 units of insulin 365 days a year will cost the patient anywhere between $18,000-$20,000. Studies show that approximately 80% of type 2 diabetes-related deaths occur in low to middle income countries. (11) Often people either cannot pay for insulin, or will suffer the complications of this powerful medication and continued eating pattern.

Insulin list prices over the last decade

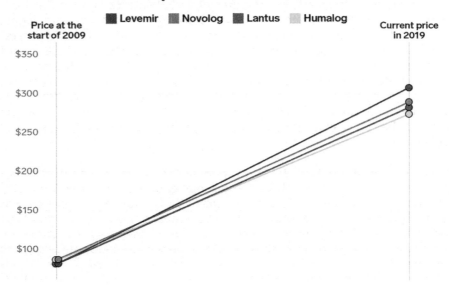

Gillett, Rachel. *One Chart Reveals How the Cost of Insulin Has Skyrocketed in the US, Even Though Nothing about It Has Changed.* 18 Sept. 2019, www.businessinsider.com/insulin-price-increased-last-decade-chart-2019-9.

I would like to introduce an analogy. For a diabetic individual, eating a consistent carbohydrate diet is the equivalent to consistently setting your house on fire via carbohydrates, then dousing the flames with a high-powered chemical extinguisher of insulin. While the house may continue to survive several fires if they are put out quickly, the effects of this type of approach will be apparent. The cabinets are burnt, the floor is destroyed, the plumbing is ruined, and the roof is obliterated. Yes, the structure may still be standing, but it is not a house I would feel safe living in. What if you have too much fire and not enough fire suppressant? What if you have only a small fire and douse the entire house with fire suppressant? Can a house really survive being set on fire and then doused with chemicals from a fire extinguisher several times a day, day-in and day-out, for years?

I'd like to propose a simple solution. How about we stop setting the house on fire in the first place?

To further understand this analogy, I would like to give you a brief overview of basic human physiology and metabolism. I want you to understand what is going on when someone is diabetic, so you can feel confident in my proposed solution.

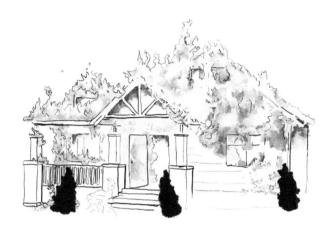

Before we move on, I would like to take a moment to validate that there are several factors outside of the foods you eat that can impact blood sugar levels. These factors include sleep quality and duration, stress, and high intensity exercise. While all these factors are relevant, my many years as a dietitian as well as the research articles cited in this book, consistently demonstrate that the *most crucial* factor for preventing and reversing diabetes is diet. In my experience, all the above variables as well as energy, focus, motivation, mental clarity, reduced pain, and an inflammatory response improve significantly when you start eating in a way that aligns with human physiology. Human physiology is how your cells, organs, and tissues were designed to function and thrive.

Let's discuss carbohydrates. Carbohydrates were an extremely small part of the diet for the majority of human evolution. Historically, we ate mostly fresh meat and fat. Humans living in artic climates could go years without consuming any plant material. Many people are surprised to hear that you do not need to eat any carbohydrates to live and thrive, and certainly not the Nutrition Pyramid's six to eleven serving suggestion of "healthy whole grains" or copious amounts of fruits and vegetables. The number of essential carbohydrates humans require is zero.

Why are we taught to consume so many carbohydrates? There is a whole chapter dedicated to discussing the current nutrition guidelines towards the end of this book. Briefly, corporate interest and profits from cheap mono-crops including corn, wheat, and soy became a big business during and after World War II. The Academy of Nutrition, which is the governing board of all dietitians and formerly called the "American Dietetic Association," is currently sponsored by Pepsi and General Mills. Pharmaceutical company and maker of diabetic drugs, GlaxoSmithKline, sponsored FNCE, the "largest annual

THE ROLE OF
MACRONUTRIENTS

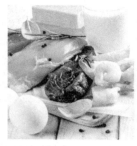 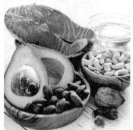 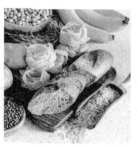

PROTEIN	FAT	CARBS
Builds + repairs tissues	Provides energy	Provides energy
Makes enzymes + hormones	Makes + balances hormones	**In the absense of carbs, the body will use fat for energy**
Transports + stores nutrients	Forms cell membranes	
ESSENTIAL	ESSENTIAL	NON-ESSENTIAL

meeting of food and nutrition experts." (12) From the day I became an RD in 2009, I have adamantly refused to be a member of the Academy of Nutrition. I firmly believe corporate sponsorship can have a profound impact on nutritional guidelines as well as the foods we are encouraged to recommend to patients.

How do other dietitians feel about the Academy's sponsors? When I brought this concern to my dietitian coworkers several years ago, no one appeared surprised or bothered. I got shrugged shoulders. "What can we do," was the prevailing message I heard. "You're not going to change the world, Michelle. You're fighting a losing battle. There's too much money at stake." While I am not naïve to think that big businesses are going to put the public health interest before the portfolios of their shareholders, I do believe complacency is complicity. The right information and the courage to act on it changed my life, and I believe it could change yours.

There is an incredible amount of money in processed carbohydrates, and I am not solely talking about the companies who produce snack foods, snack bars, candy, and "healthy whole grain" products. The top three

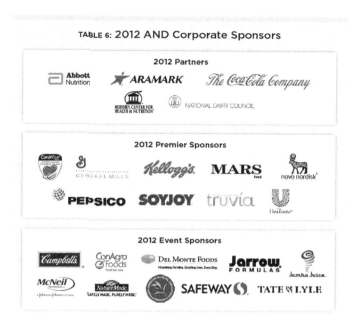

TABLE 6: 2012 AND Corporate Sponsors

Academy Sponsors from 2012. Credit: Nestle, Marion, and Michael Pollan. *Food Politics: How the Food Industry Influences Nutrition and Health*. University of California Press, 2013.

pharmaceutical companies in the United States reported 2019 earnings between 5-10 billion dollars. (13) There is no entity that loves the phrase, "Eat carbohydrates and sugar in moderation," more than the pharmaceutical industry. They are making *a lot of money* producing medications that treat the diseases caused by the overconsumption of carbohydrates. The concept of "moderation" is encouraged by dietitians, doctors, and mental health care providers alike. You are unlikely to go through most food bloggers or health coaches' Instagram feeds without seeing someone telling you to "Go ahead and eat the ice cream. Just eat it in moderation." As you will see throughout this book, moderation with processed carbohydrates is not possible on a physiological basis. In fact, carbohydrates, specifically processed carbohydrates, have been shown in studies to have the same qualities as addictive substances. (14)

Consuming processed carbohydrates is a dangerous game, and the American public is losing. It has been estimated that dramatically shifting our current diet to reduce or eliminate processed carbohydrates could put the top three producers of packaged foods and insulin out of business within three to five years. Since carbohydrates are a main contributor to most chronic disease, and diabetic drugs earn CEOs billions of dollars per year, do not expect nutrition guidelines to change any time soon.

In a person with or without diabetes, consuming any carbohydrate, such as a piece of bread, an apple, a breakfast cereal, or potato chips, causes a rise in blood sugar.

In non-diabetics, insulin is produced by the pancreas. After carbohydrates are eaten and they enter the blood stream, causing a rise in blood glucose, the pancreas releases insulin to shuttle carbohydrates to cells in the body.

In some individuals with diabetes, the pancreas no longer produces any insulin. Without insulin to bring blood sugar levels back down, a person with diabetes will have high blood glucose levels after carbohydrates are consumed. In other individuals with diabetes, the pancreas only produces a small amount of insulin. If these individuals consume carbohydrates, blood glucose levels will be reduced somewhat, but they will still be above the normal range. Finally, some individuals with diabetes produce insulin, but their cells are now resistant to the insulin. This means the insulin cannot shuttle the blood glucose where it needs to go. All of these scenarios result in elevated blood glucose which over time causes the many determinantal complications associated with diabetes.

Sample graph of a person's blood glucose level with type 2 diabetes who still produces some insulin versus someone without diabetes. Both individuals consumed the same meal with the same amount of carbohydrates.

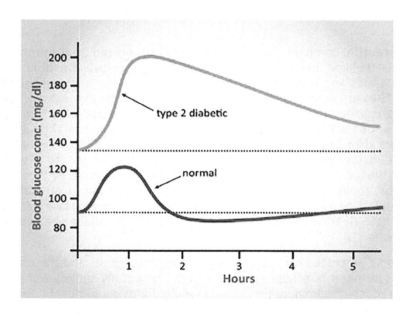

Graph of glucose monitor of a type 2 diabetic who no longer produces any insulin. This person ate a banana at 4:45pm.

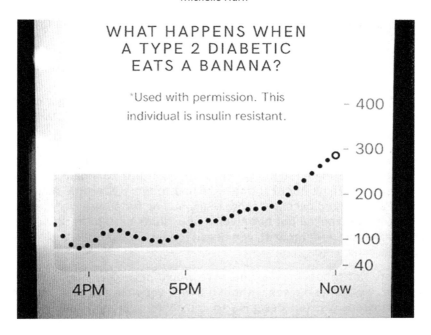

One of the most important factors in preventing diabetes is to keep insulin levels low. In order to reverse diabetes, we want to do the same thing, keep insulin low and re-sensitize cells to insulin's effects. (15)

Eating carbohydrates such as fruit, bread, pasta, or oatmeal **increases** blood glucose and insulin levels. Reducing, or minimizing carbohydrates **decreases** blood glucose and insulin levels. Knowing that carbohydrates are not essential for heath, and understanding that reducing them can decrease high blood glucose levels and potentially reverse diabetes, does it make sense for health professionals to recommend a low-carbohydrate way of eating?

Currently, a low-carbohydrate way of eating is not the prevailing nutritional advice from most dietitians, doctors, and health professionals. The consensus continues to be that diabetics should eat lots of fruits and vegetables as well as whole grains. Some professionals even think it is acceptable for diabetics to consume sugar "in moderation." Recall that fruits, vegetables, whole grains, and sugar cause blood sugar to rise and require insulin. If a diabetic can obtain all of our nutrition from foods that do not cause this detrimental rise in blood sugar, it makes sense that we should explore this option.

Here are some questions I would like to address. I am not sure that we do a good job of explaining these points to our diabetic patients in the acute care hospital or outpatient setting. You may find these questions and answers helpful if you or someone you know has diabetes or prediabetes.

- 1. If my blood sugar is high and I take a prescription insulin, where does the sugar in my blood go?
- 2. What does it mean to have "excellent" blood sugar control?
- 3. Are there potential consequences or side effects for a type 2 diabetic that uses insulin over the long term?

Hyperglycemia, which is high blood sugar, happens when either the pancreas is no longer secreting enough insulin, or the cells are no longer sensitive to insulin's effects. Think about a time you had to work overtime at your job. You were a solid employee and were really pulling for a raise, so you worked your tail off and cranked out two twelve-hour shifts back-to-back. At the end of the second twelve-hour shift, you began to fantasize about sleep. You were completely exhausted.

Humans are not robots or machines. We would never ask a human to work 12 hours a day, 7 days a week without a break, yet we ask this of our pancreas. The pancreas was not designed to constantly secrete insulin. When we consume foods that are very high in carbohydrates and sugars, day in and day out, overtime we put tremendous stress on our pancreas. Most humans consume highly processed carbohydrates, sugars, and whole food carbohydrate sources several times a day, every day, 365 days a year.

What if your boss asked you to work twelve hour shifts 365 days a year? You would likely experience a physical or mental breakdown. This is what is happening to the pancreas of someone who becomes diabetic. The pancreas is exhausted, and it desperately needs a vacation day.

I would like you to present you with a second analogy. Look at the cartoon of a hoarder's house below. There are boxes and bags spread all over the house and old newspapers are stacked to the ceiling. Trash is scattered over the lawn and clothes are spewing out the windows. You can't walk through the front door because it's blockaded by too much junk. There is no room left for any more items. *This is what is happening in the body of a diabetic.* The muscles are so full of glycogen, or stored sugar, that the extra sugar goes to the liver. The liver becomes packed with sugar and there just isn't any more room at the inn! In fact, it is not uncommon for individuals with diabetes to experience non-alcoholic fatty liver disease. All the excess sugar over time can actually damage the liver. (16)

What makes sense to do in this situation? In this scenario, it seems to make sense to get rid of some of the excess stuff (stored carbohydrates) and stop bringing in more stuff (new carbohydrates). It is time to burn up some of that stored muscle and liver glycogen. This can be done by engaging in some form of exercise like going for a brisk walk. By replacing carbohydrates with

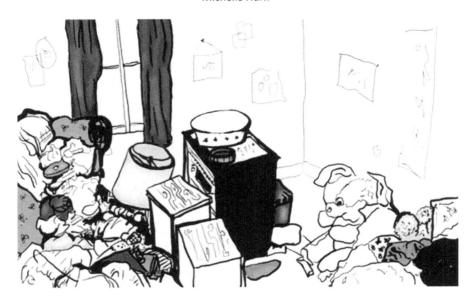

protein and fat, a diabetic can easily become insulin sensitive, instead of re-sistant, over a relatively short period of time. In fact, a study done on obese patients showed a 75% increase in insulin sensitivity after a mere *14 days on a low-carbohydrate diet.* (17)

Unfortunately, many people faced with a diagnosis of diabetes are encouraged to continue eating carbohydrates and simply take medications to manage the negative effects caused by carbohydrates. If consuming carbohydrates caused the initial problem, it seems a fair question to ask if consuming carbohydrates is the best solution.

One potential issue with blood glucose lowering medication is the side effects. In my experience, many patients continue to eat carbohydrates and proceed to start taking blood glucose lowering medications, often metformin and then insulin. The most common side effects of metformin are dizziness, nausea, diarrhea and weakness. One of insulin's side effects is weight gain. (18)

When a patient takes insulin, it forces glucose out of the blood. Where does it go? Remember the analogy of the hoarder's house. There is no room left to store the blood glucose in the muscles or liver. While our bodies have a relatively small capacity to store sugar or glucose, our bodies have a virtually *unlimited ability to store fat*. If glucose cannot be stored as muscle or liver glycogen, *it will be stored as fat*. Since we know high blood sugar is poten-tially dangerous, is it less dangerous to get the sugar out of the bloodstream even if it is stored as fat? It depends. It could potentially be much more dangerous.

When it comes to body fat, you have two types, subcutaneous fat and visceral fat. Subcutaneous fat is the visible fat under your skin. Visceral fat is stored within the abdominal cavity and around a number of important internal organs such as the liver, pancreas, and intestines. Depending on your genetics, you may store more or less total fat as visceral fat. The more fat you store as visceral, the greater chance you have of complications such as a heart attack or stroke. It is important to note that the sugar in your blood does not magically disappear into an alternative universe when you take insulin or other oral diabetic medications. It gets stored as fat, and it can potentially lead to a heart attack, stroke, or systemic inflammation (19).

What does it mean to have, "excellent blood sugar control"? I recently came across a doctor's note on a diabetic patient. This particular patient had a large wound that was not healing well, high blood pressure, stomach ulcers, high triglycerides, and was a type 2 diabetic. The doctor wrote, "Patient has excellent glycemic (blood sugar) control." This patient was taking over 100 units of insulin daily while eating more than 250 grams of carbohydrates a day. I would like to question what exactly is "excellent" about this scenario?

Continuing to eat in a way that requires medication and prolongs illness when there is a sustainable, health promoting alternative seems backward. Ultimately, it should be up to the patient to decide which course of action they want to pursue, medication or changing the foods they eat. It is my view that patients have a right to understand their options.

If you have never had the opportunity to spend much time in a hospital, consider yourself lucky. Most of the patients I see are so profoundly overly fat and under muscled that they cannot walk the few steps to the hospital bathroom. Incontinence of bladder and bowel in patients under the age of 50 is relatively common. In fact, urinary incontinence is 70% higher in diabetics than in the general population. (20) Hyperglycemia, which is high blood sugar, prevents wounds from healing. (21) I have seen wounds so massive, infected, and oozing with pus, that the medical staff utilized maggot therapy. Google it if you dare; it still makes my stomach queasy! Over 50% of the patients I see in an acute care setting have diabetes. Many of them have irreversible consequences from the years of damage done by unmanaged high blood sugar.

What does a diabetic's diet look like? It hurts my soul to see the meals fed to patients in a hospital setting. Not surprisingly, these are the same type of foods that are recommended outside the hospital setting. Recall that most diabetics are put on "consistent carbohydrate" diets. This ensures they have a certain number of carbohydrates per meal. Here is an example of what a patient might receive on a diabetic diet in a hospital setting:

Breakfast:

- 2 whole wheat pancakes
- Margarine
- Sugar-free maple syrup
- Apple slices
- 2% milk
- Hash browns
- Nonfat vanilla yogurt
- Coffee with and no-sugar substitute

Calories: 738
Carbohydrates: 89 grams
Sugar: 48 grams
Protein: 27 grams
Fat: 30 grams

Lunch:

- Grilled cheese (2 oz cheese) on whole wheat bread
- Tomato basil soup
- 1 small bag potato chips
- 4 ounces grape juice
- Low-sugar chocolate pudding

Calories: 685
Carbohydrates: 88 grams
Sugar: 25 grams
Protein: 16 grams
Fat: 28 grams

Dinner:

- Roast turkey (3 ounces) and gravy
- Mashed potatoes and gravy
- 1-piece whole wheat toast
- Steamed green beans
- 4 ounces diced peaches in light syrup
- 2% milk
- Low-sugar vanilla pudding

Calories: 662
Carbohydrates: 88 grams
Sugar: 30 grams
Protein: 33 grams
Fat: 20 grams

Totals: Calories: 2058
Carbohydrates: 265 grams (52%)
Sugar: 103 grams (25.75 teaspoons of sugar for a diabetic!)
Protein: 76 grams (14%)
Fat: 78 grams (34%

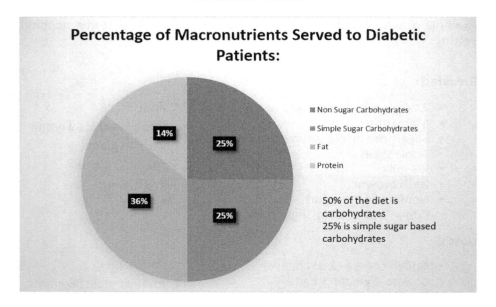

Percentage of Macronutrients Served to Diabetic Patients:

- Non Sugar Carbohydrates
- Simple Sugar Carbohydrates
- Fat
- Protein

50% of the diet is carbohydrates
25% is simple sugar based carbohydrates

14% 25% 36% 25%

Our human physiology was designed to run quite well on meat and fat. Throughout our evolution, carbohydrates were quite rare. Vegetables and fruits were much smaller and had less sugar content than today's varieties. During winters or prolonged periods of heat, it was not unusual for humans to go months without taking in any fruits or vegetables. It was not until approximately 8,000 years ago, due to the rise of agriculture, humans began to have easy access to things like wheat, grains, and green vegetables. In the last 50 years, our access to highly palatable, refined carbohydrate foods has become completely ubiquitous. It is challenging to go anywhere and not be confronted with some type of high-carbohydrate, sugar-laden treat. I took my dog to the veterinarian and was immediately offered a free mocha from a coffee machine. I needed to pick up an air filter at Home Depot, and as I approached the check-out stand, my eyes fell on soda and candy bars. Every gas station, grocery store, and hospital offer sugary treats for clients and patients alike. Anyone who works in health care will note that free donuts and pastries are often brought into the break rooms to share.

But surely, we need *some* carbohydrates for energy, right?

The human body does not require any carbohydrates to survive and thrive. Please note that I am not "anti-carbohydrate," as some people do very well with a small amount of carbohydrates in their diets. For individuals dealing with obesity, diabetes, heart disease, autoimmune disorders, and food addictions, which are real and should be taken seriously, it can be beneficial to remove carbohydrates from your diet for a specific period of time. It may prove invaluable in your healing process.

For many people, highly processed, high sugar containing, carbohydrate-based foods, such as cookies, cereal, or bread, have become powerful coping mechanisms for dealing with trauma or stress. It may be helpful to seek support from a medical professional to deal with difficult emotions when changing your diet.

Your body does an excellent job of producing all the carbohydrates it needs through proteins, glycerol, and lactate. Under normal conditions, your body can get all the glucose required to function optimally through a process called gluconeogenesis. (22) That's a fancy word, but let's break it down:

- Gluco: glucose
- Neo: new
- Genesis: creates

The word gluconeogenesis simply means *to create new glucose*. In fact, out of the three main macronutrients (carbohydrates, fat and protein*), the only macronutrient we can survive without is carbohydrates.*

The pancreas does release insulin when you eat protein, but it is significantly less than when you consume carbohydrates. The small insulin response after you eat something like a steak or chicken breast has been shown to have no negative effects on our system. In fact, insulin allows protein to keep blood glucose stable via gluconeogenesis. The rest of the broken-down protein that is not used to produce new glucose can participate in essential roles in the human body. While protein is important for muscle growth, it has many functions. Protein acts as enzymes, rebuilds muscle tissue, participates in cell-to-cell communication, immune function, collagen production, becomes precursors to neurotransmitters, and participates in digestion and hormone production.

It is almost as if our bodies were *designed to use protein for needed glucose instead of processed carbohydrates.* Protein has all the benefits and none of the detriments. Yes, you can absolutely eat carbohydrates for fuel, but for many people there is a high price to pay in the way of poor health in the long run.

You might be wondering, *What about "healthy" whole grains, and fruits and vegetables? Where do those fit in?* We will cover fruits, vegetables, and whole grains in depth in our chapter, Plants vs Animals, so keep reading.

Is it as simple as just eating protein? Can you simply invest in eating lots of grilled chicken and restore your health? No, you cannot. *The human body requires fat.* Dietary fat has gotten a bad reputation thanks to flawed, bias research by many self-serving organizations and specifically by Ancel Keys. Keys, an American physiologist, worked to find data that would link certain foods people were eating to heart disease. It was his hypothesis that animal products, especially those high in saturated fat, such as butter, cheese, and high-fat meat, caused heart disease and other chronic issues. While analyzing the dietary patterns of 22 countries, he was unable to link the majority of countries' saturated fat intake to heart disease. Statistically, there was no significant correlation between meat and saturated fat consumption and the prevalence heart disease.

Instead of forgoing his hypothesis, in his report, he decided to only use seven countries and leave out the other fifteen that did not fit his hypothesis. In fact, of the 15 countries he left out of his report, several of them *ate the highest amount of animal products and had the least amount of heart disease.* He skewed his research by only showing a percentage of his results. (23)

Due in part to Ancel Keys' hypothesis and low-fat advocacy, we have paid a high price with our dietary recommendations and subsequent obesity crisis. In the 1980s, the first round of the dietary recommendations was released. Check out the chart below to see how obesity has shifted since their release. To this day, many people are afraid to eat fat despite it being an essential macronutrient for health.

Prevalence of Obesity among US Adults

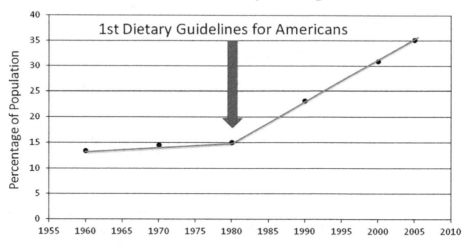

Picture Credit: "CDC - NCHS - National Center for Health Statistics." *Centers for Disease Control and Prevention*, Centers for Disease Control and Prevention, 7 Aug. 2020, www.cdc.gov/nchs/index.htm

The brain is the fattiest organ in the body, comprised of 60% fat. There is sufficient evidence to suggest that children who do not receive adequate fat in those first crucial years of life can have significant cognitive impairments due to inadequate myelination of nerve cells in the brain. (24)

Fat is an important energy source. How much fat can a human store? A lot! While the human body can only store about 2,000 calories of carbohydrates (you may have heard of a marathon runner "bonking" or "hitting the wall" after running out of carbohydrates) it can store more than 100,000 calories of fat. Fat is an important part of our cells, and it plays a role in blood clotting, wound healing, and inflammation. Fat is the carrier for fat-soluble vitamins A, D, E, and K. It promotes satiety and assists in keeping blood sugar stable. Is an animal based, high-fat diet safe? Has anyone ever followed a high-meat, high-fat diet for an extended period of time?

Allow me to segue into the topic of an explorer named Vilhjalmur Stefansson. Stefansson was an Icelandic explorer and ethnologist. Ethnology is the branch of anthropology that analyzes characteristics of different peoples and the relationships between them. Stefansson lived with the Inuit Eskimos for years at a time. He was amazed at their incredible health and lack of disease. He would later go on the document his experience stating that the Inuit diet consisted of "90% meat" and would often "eat nothing but meat and fish for 6-9 months of the year." He found that he and his fellow explorers of European and South Sea Island descent were also perfectly healthy on such a diet. Many people at the time balked at the idea that an all-meat diet could possibly be a sustainable, healthy diet for most humans.

At this point Stefansson had his personal, anecdotal experience. He had followed an all-meat diet for many months at a time over a four-year period with no ill effects. In fact, in his writings, he states he felt "better than ever." He also had the opportunity to live amongst the Inuit Eskimos and witness them thriving off this type of diet. He did not just survey them and ask what they were eating; he hunted, ate, and lived with them. Still, he used this experience to create a hypothesis.

Stefansson's hypothesis stated that as long as significant fat was consumed, and all meat diet was healthy for humans. He also believed that this type of diet was to be followed without calorie restriction. The person should eat meat and fat until satiated. Mind you, this was before the big cereal, granola bar, and bread companies were around to throw a fit.

Stefansson was so passionate about this way of eating that he volunteered an entire year of his life to undergo an experiment to prove its effectiveness. Stefansson and his fellow explorer, Karsten Anderson, agreed to undertake a study to demonstrate that they could eat a 100% meat diet in a closely observed laboratory setting for the first several weeks. For the rest of the year, paid observers followed them to ensure dietary compliance.

There were no nutrient deficiencies, and the two men remained perfectly healthy. Their bowels remained normal, except that their stools were smaller. Stefansson's gingivitis disappeared. During this experiment, his intake had varied between 2,000 and 3,100 calories per day, and he derived an average of almost eighty percent of his energy from animal fat and roughly twenty percent from protein. Daily intake varied from 100-140 grams of protein, 200-300 grams of fat, and 7-12 grams of carbohydrates. (26)

Stefansson summarized the results of his study in his book, *The Fat of the Land*, "Meat, as some have contended is a particularly stimulating food, which I verified during our New York experiment to the extent that it seems to me I was more optimistic and energetic than ordinarily. I looked forward with more anticipation to the next day or next job and was more likely to expect pleasure or success. We now add the suggestion that the optimism may be directly caused by what they (Eskimos) eat." (27) He went on to state, "a phase of our experiment has a relation to slimming, slenderizing, reducing, the treatment of obesity. I was about ten pounds overweight at the beginning of the meat diet and lost all of it." (27)

Have you ever heard of this individual or this study? I had not heard of Stefansson until I researched a low-carbohydrate, animal-based way of eating. Being such a profound success, why is this year-long experiment not discussed in medical circles? Unfortunately, money is a driving force in health care. There is very little money in restoring health or expediting death. In health care, money is made by keeping people perpetually sick and dependent on medications, surgeries, and consistent hospital visits.

I have heard several medical providers express concern over a high-meat, high-fat, low-carbohydrate diet. There is a lot of fearmongering around the subjects of meat and fat. An article published by the Diabetes Research Institute boldly claims, "Despite the evidence that reducing carbohydrate lowers body weight and, in patients with type two diabetes, improves glucose control, few data are available about sustainability, safety, and efficacy in the long term." (28)

Another article states, "Studies in the literature are indeed controversial, possibly because these diets are generally poorly defined; this, together with the intrinsic complexity of dietary interventions, makes it difficult to compare results from different studies." (29)

Despite the overwhelming evidence that a low-carbohydrate, high-fat, moderate protein diet is effective for diabetics, nutrition recommendations remain unchanged.

Can you eat a high-carbohydrate, low-fat diet, and be metabolically healthy? Yes, it is possible. Some people, including endurance athletes, eat very high amounts of carbohydrates, small amounts of low-fat protein, and they keep overall fat intake low. Many of these individuals claim to be in excellent health, and some have impressive endurance performances.

While some people seem to be able to consume carbohydrates, including processed carbohydrates, without any apparent issues, my research and experience has shown me that these people represent the minority. For many people, carbohydrates create a cycle (pictured below) that includes eating carbohydrates, creating high blood sugar, causing an insulin response that pushes blood sugar towards fat storage, then, experiencing blood sugar crashes which leads to carbohydrate cravings. Have you ever had a bagel and coffee at 8 AM, only to wonder why you are craving a donut or granola bar at 10 AM? A high-carbohydrate, low-fat way of eating can create a vicious cycle.

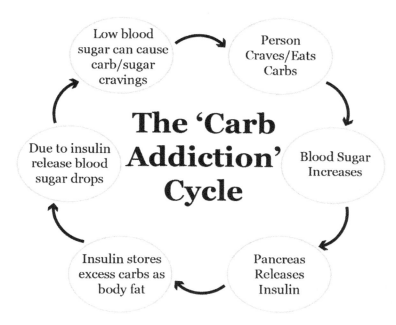

Another potential pitfall of a high-carbohydrate, low-fat way of eating is that it might be inadequate in the essential fatty acids needed to support mental health and allow the brain to recover from stress. We will dive into this issue in our next chapter.

Perhaps the fact that *most diets are failing is not because humans are lazy and weak.* Perhaps the current dietary regimen that causes blood sugar spikes, blood sugar crashes, increasing stress hormones, and subsequent hunger is setting people up to fail. If you remember nothing else from this book, please underline the following sentences: Insulin suppresses fatty acid oxidation and stimulates fat deposition. This is a fancy way of saying insulin prevents your body from being able to burn your excess fat and it allows your body to store even more fat. This means you can exercise and count calories until the cows come home, but ***if you are activating insulin by eating too many***

carbohydrates, you will be unable to reduce the amount of fat you have on your body.

Throughout this book, we will continue to look at evidence to support that the foundation of health comes from an animal-based, high-fat, moderate protein, low-carbohydrate based diet. The amount of plants to include in your diet is more nuanced and varies depending on tolerance, goals, and current state of health.

Finally, a peer reviewed study states, "The severity of the diabetes epidemic warrants careful and renewed consideration of our assumptions about the diet for diabetes. By reducing carbohydrates in the diet, we have been able to taper patients off as much as 150 units of insulin per day in 8 days, with marked improvement in glycemic control-even normalization of glycemic parameters." (30) Carbohydrate restriction is the single most effective intervention when it comes to reducing all the features of metabolic syndrome. (30) That is a sentence worth reading again.

A significant barrier to implementing a low-carbohydrate diet is the traditional fear that there will be a negative effect on blood lipids. For example, some people point to the tendency of dietary saturated fat to raise blood total cholesterol. (31, 32) The line of thinking is, "If I eat saturated fat, I will raise my total cholesterol. If I raise my cholesterol and specifically LDL, I will have heart disease."

Eating a high amount of saturated fat did not cause heart disease through 3.5 million years of evolution. We added carbohydrates to our diet, and now we have heart disease. I will delve deeper into the relationship between carbohydrates, insulin resistance, and LDL in my chapter on heart disease. You will discover how diabetes and heart disease are closely related. (33) They share a common culprit, which I bet you'll be able to identify soon if you haven't already.

Low-carbohydrate diets continue to demonstrate that they have little risk and good overall compliance. At the same time, the monumental failure of the low-fat paradigm to meet expectations, coupled with the continuing report of side effects of various drugs, indicates a *past due need* to reevaluate the role of reduction of carbohydrates in diabetic therapy.

My goal for this chapter was for you to start thinking about the nutrition recommendations for diabetes in a different light. You have the power to completely change your course of treatment by shifting the foods you choose to eat. If this chapter made you angry, that is probably a good thing as it means you are thinking critically. If you or someone you love has been suffering needlessly, a change in eating habits could be an important step towards healing.

Amber Wentworth

Email: lonestarketogirl@gmail.com
Instagram: @LoneStarKetoGirl
Twitter: @Lone_Star_Keto
Facebook: Lone Star Keto
TikTok: @lonestarketogirl
YouTube: LoneStarKeto
Website: Lone-Star-Keto.com
Carnivore and Fasting Coaching: https://meatrx.com/product/amber-w/

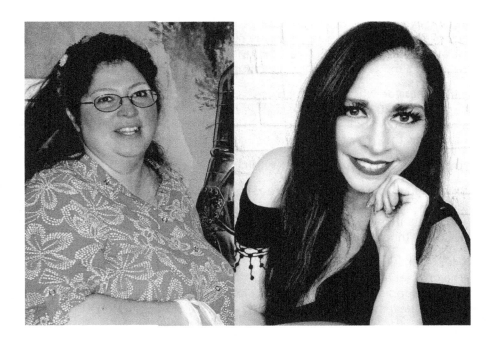

My name is Amber. I'm 54, married, and have 2 adult kids and one granddaughter.

I've battled with weight issues since I was 10 years old. That's over 40 years! Not to mention dealing with multiple eating/exercise disorders. I've tried pretty much every diet out there at some point, including a medically supervised one at the age of 16. I've lost 80-100lbs four times. Three were via Weight Watchers with the same exact results-gaining all or most of it back, sometimes more. Gotta love the low-fat, high-carb, processed food-filled Standard American Diet.

At my heaviest I was over 240 lbs. and wore a size 26. That's pretty major considering I'm only 5'2". My health suffered horribly as well. I became hypertensive (210/110) and pre-diabetic. At one point, I was taking 4 medications for my high BP. I had major acid reflux and took Nexium every day for 8 years. My rosacea was severe and a great embarrassment. It was bad enough I was huge, but to have my face look like Rudolph with acne as well was downright degrading. I had digestive issues that caused me great pain. Also, I had Reynaud's Syndrome. I was a health mess.

But even worse than the physical pain was the emotional and psychological pain I endured. I was depressed and spent a good 20 years of my life hiding from the world. I became a spectator of my own life. Watching on the sidelines instead of living. Even after losing the weight those 3 times, I knew in the back of my mind there was no way I could sustain that way of living for the rest of my life. I was miserable--always hungry, angry, and feeling deprived. It was just a matter of time until the weight came piling back on. And it did.

All that changed when I stumbled across the Keto Diet. I started my keto journey in July of 2017. To say it was a life-changer is a huge understatement. I knew the first week I had found a gold mine. I told my husband that I could live like this the rest of my life and be happy. That was HUGE!

I started to research and read everything I could get my hands on.

Along the keto journey, I was able to get off Nexium and 3 of my blood pressure meds. My stomach issues and rosacea greatly improved, I lost 80-ish lbs. in 8 months, and my depression was gone. I was also able to maintain my weight loss longer than I ever had without any worry I wouldn't be able to sustain it.

Since I still had a little healing to do and a friend kept pestering me to give the carnivore diet a try, I transitioned into it March 2019. I'm now off ALL medications and supplements. I have zero stomach issues and the rosacea is almost gone! I've never felt better.

I am not dogmatic when it comes to the "right" way to do keto/carnivore. I believe we all have to figure out what works for us and what we can sustain. After all, this is not a temporary diet. If you can't stick with it, what's the point?

One thing I've noticed in the keto/carnivore community is so many focus on the weight loss aspect. I get it. I did, too. However, since I've experienced true health, I now look at weight loss as a great side effect. Not the whole story. I know it's easier said than done, but when you focus on health, great things happen!! Patience is key!!!

I used to think back on the past and feel great sadness for all I missed out on. But now I think of it as preparing me to be able to relate and help others. And if I can inspire just one person to make positive health changes and not have to suffer like I did, then everything I do is worth it!

Mary Roberts

Email: mary@ketovangelist.com
Facebook: KetoMary71
Instagram: @ketomary71
Coaching: https://ketogeniclifestylecoaching.com/coaches/mary-roberts/

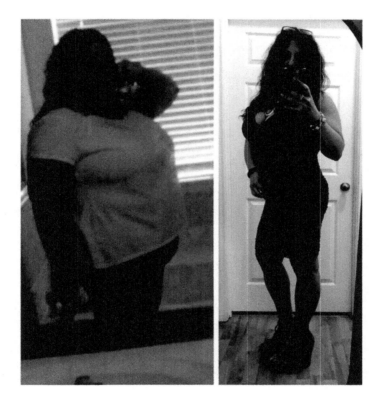

After battling my weight from my preteen years to age 42, I decided to pursue a ketogenic way of eating. It took me 22 months to lose 106 pounds and I've been maintaining for over 4 years now.

In addition to losing weight, I reversed my type 2 diabetes and returned my blood pressure to normal. I'm not on any medications anymore for either of those issues. I also no longer have asthma/allergy issues, no more sleep apnea, no more snoring, no new psoriasis breakouts, no more depression or fatigue and I've only been sick with a minor cold twice in over 6 years that I've been eating this way.

Most importantly I have found food sobriety/recovery from my disordered eating. I am over six years food sober and I have a passion for helping other people get free from the obsession with food and overcoming food/carb addiction.

I offer one-on-one coaching and specialty groups. My most popular group is the Food Addiction and Recovery group.

Elizabeth Ping

Type 1 Diabetic

Instagram: @diabadassbeth

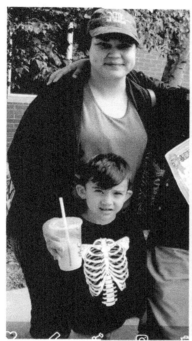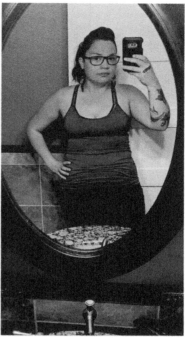

On June 5, 2016 my life changed forever! At the age of 29, I was diagnosed with type 1 diabetes.

This diagnosis was a huge curveball for me, and I found it difficult to adjust. Six months after the diagnosis, I started my keto journey because my husband suggested it. I followed the ketogenic diet sporadically until 2020. For me, I found I didn't really enjoy it because there was a lot of math involved to do it the proper way.

I felt I already had enough math to do to manage my type 1 diabetes. I wanted to find something easier. On March 1, 2020, I started a carnivore diet. It didn't take long to see results with my improved blood sugars, and after a month, I started to see more results, like weight loss, more energy, and great skin. I prefer this diet because it's super easy. I just eat when hungry, and I stop when I'm satisfied. I'm down so much in insulin usage, and I get spectacular blood sugars! I save a ton of money monthly on insulin and diabetic supplies! I am a true believer in this diet because I feel amazing. I don't even feel diabetic.

It feels like some doctors want you to cripple yourself with the standard diet. This will cause you use more insulin and spend more money just to stay alive! It's a vicious cycle. You can make the change and become a believer like me.

Chapter 2

Mental Illness: Healing with Food

Mental illness has a long history of being stigmatized and misunderstood in our society. A study conducted in 2002 to determine attitudes towards individuals with mental illnesses demonstrated that medical students, as well as the general public, tend to believe that individuals with mental illness, "had a peculiar and stereotypical appearance." The study went on to find that most study participants stated they would, "prefer that facilities for psychiatric care be located away from the community." (1)

Mental illness tends to be divided into two categories. In the first category, you have the individuals struggling with anxiety and depression. The general consensus for these individuals is that they can completely recover and live normal, productive lives. Unfortunately, there is still a stigma that recovering from depression or severe anxiety is as simple as "thinking positively," "not being so lazy," or simply "getting your act together."

In the second category, you have the individuals dealing with disorders such as bi-polar disorder, schizophrenia, and schizoaffective disorder. These people tend to be deemed as "really crazy" or "beyond help." Often the goal of the medical community is to simply manage the symptoms of these difficult to treat mental illnesses. Having worked in several psychiatric facilities, I have witnessed the attitudes of many medical professionals when it comes to dealing with illnesses such as schizophrenia or unmanaged bi-polar disorder. While there are certainly exceptions, many believe that these types of mental illnesses require a person to live in a monitored facility while being highly medicated for the remainder of their lives. The dogma is, "There is no cure, so we manage the symptoms."

While I would like to think our society's attitude towards individuals struggling with debilitating mental illness is evolving to displaying compassion and empathy, our ability to effectively treat mental illnesses is woefully lacking. While medications, talk therapy, and lifestyle management can provide some relief, they often address the symptoms of mental illness instead at looking at the root causes of the disease.

It has been suggested that mental illness is increasing at an exponential rate. Is this really true, or are we just over-diagnosing or "diagnosing everything" these days? It is a fair question. As the stigma associated with mental illness begins to subside and access to treatment increases, it would certainly make sense that we would see more mental health diagnoses.

In a recent interview, Dr. Chris Palmer, a Harvard-trained psychiatrist, was asked if his research showed that the increase in mental health diagnoses was simply related to the decreasing stigma of mental disorders. Are there more people developing mental illnesses or are the people who had been struggling with mental illnesses for many years just now seeking help and being diagnosed?

Before answering, Dr. Palmer noted several additional hypotheses for the increase in diagnoses of mental illness.

One hypothesis he hears frequently is, "society sucks." Stress, society in general, and everyone being attached to their cell phones, are thought to contribute to the declining mental health of our nation. I would certainly agree that having a face-to-face conversation is becoming increasingly rare. It reminds me of my experience treating a young patient at a psychiatric facility where I was the lead dietitian. She was eating poorly due to severe depression. When discussing social support, she paused, stared directly at me and stated, "I have over 500 Facebook friends and no one to call when I'm sad."

Could it be that isolation, stress, and loneliness are the main factors contributing to an increase in mental illness?

Dr. Palmer does not think so. He also does not believe that a push for antidepressants from the pharmaceutical industry is the main reason we are seeing an exponential increase in mental illnesses diagnoses. He wrapped up his thoughts by stating a firm, "no, it's not," when asked again if the decrease in stigma was the main driver for seeing an increase in cases being diagnosed.

He recognizes that prescription medication companies, lack of social interactions and our recent campaign to destigmatize anxiety, depression, bullying, and suicidal ideation have certainly played a role in the increase of mental health diagnosis. (2) He believes we are asking the wrong question when it comes to explaining the increasing numbers of mental illnesses.

What's causing the mental disorder in the first place?

While writing this book, I started a YouTube Channel. Currently, I have interviewed over two dozen individuals. Every single individual I interviewed admitted, many candidly, to dealing with anxiety, depression, or feeling of hopelessness and worthlessness. Several of the individuals I interviewed discussed feeling so low that they fixated on thoughts around taking their own lives. Having personally dealt with severe, debilitating depression, I became curious about the root cause of mental illness.

Mental illness is *increasing rapidly* in the United States. It is truly an epidemic. Approximately 13% of the United States population is taking an antidepressant. (3) Major depression is now the number one cause of disability worldwide. (4) Major depression causes more people to not be able to go to work than car accidents, cancer diagnoses, strokes, or complications from heart failure or diabetes. Anxiety disorders are up 30% in adults over the last 2 decades. In the last 15 years, the rate of bipolar disorder has doubled in adults. In the last ten years, the rate of bipolar disorder in children and adolescents has increased 4,000%. (5)

What about suicide? I have known four people who have taken their own lives. All of these individuals were bright, thoughtful, and intelligent. Tragically, they were unable to cope with severe, debilitating depression and feelings of

Suicide is the third-leading killer of people age 15-24

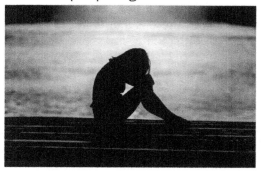

Depression is the leading cause of disability worldwide

profound hopelessness and worthlessness. Could it be that something went awry in their brains that made them more susceptible to deciding, perhaps subconsciously, to take their own lives?

Suicide rates in the United States are up 26% across the board over the last decade. For reference, in 2008 approximately 98 people died per day from suicide. (6) In 2018, 132 individuals took their lives each day. Deaths of despair, which includes suicide and deaths from an overdose, such as an opioid or alcohol overdose, are up 100% over the last decade.

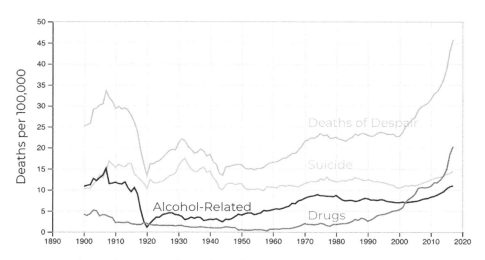

Source: Social Capital Project analyses of CDC data.

Those statistics are staggering. Is there any other health epidemic happening in this country at the same time? Could the deterioration of physical health be related to the spike in cases of mental illness?

As shown in the table below, there is a dramatic disparity in life expectancy between individuals living with mental illness and the general population. Today, people with major mental disorders live approximately 25-30 years less compared to the general population. *People with mental disorders are losing about a third of the average person's lifespan.*

Average Life Expectancy: Absence of Mental Illness	79 years
Average Life Expectancy: Person Diagnosed with Mental Illness	49–54 years

*Statistics from Metabolic Syndrome and Mental Illness by John W Newcomer MD

It is well established that individuals experiencing a mental illness face a myriad of challenges, including reduced access to health care and housing, as well as financial challenges including difficulty obtaining and maintaining employment. While all these factors may contribute to a lower quality of life and early death, the number one reason for reduced life span for those who have a major mental illness is cardiovascular (heart) disease. (7) As we will see in our chapter on heart disease, insulin resistance is a major risk factor for hardening of the arteries. As this chapter unfolds, we will look at the connection between mental illness and insulin resistance. We will answer the following question: *Why are individuals with mental illness potentially more prone to experiencing high blood sugar and insulin resistance, which can lead to heart disease?*

Statistically, the general public is not exactly the definition of healthy. As stated earlier, 70% of the United States population is either overweight or obese and an estimated 88% have some degree of metabolic dysfunction such as elevated blood sugar. Patients with major mental illnesses have an increased likelihood of diabetes, obesity, and high blood pressure compared to the general population. (8)

In 2006, the Annals of Clinical Psychiatry reported that patients with mental illness were twice as likely to have metabolic syndrome versus individuals without mental illness. (9)

Why are individuals with mental disorders significantly more likely to have heart disease, hypertension, obesity, or type 2 diabetes? It is possible that many mental illnesses are linked to errors in metabolism?

Metabolism is defined as, "The chemical processes that occur within an organism to maintain life." Simply put, metabolism is how your body breaks down the foods you eat, including carbohydrates, proteins, and fats. Metabolism allows you to have energy so you can function.

Recent studies conducted with individuals diagnosed with schizophrenia, bipolar disorder, and major depression were able to demonstrate that the brains of these individuals were unable to metabolize certain macronutrients effectively. (10) If you cannot metabolize macronutrients (proteins, carbohydrates, fats) then your brain cannot work properly. The authors of the study note that decreased phosphocreatine and ATP production have been reported in patients with psychiatric disorders. (11) The lack of phosphocreatine and ATP in the brains of these individuals demonstrates impaired energy production and a possible impaired ability to break down carbohydrates. (12,13)

As you saw in our chapter on diabetes, the body is complex. When we fuel the body with optimal, highly absorbable nutrition, it does an excellent job of keeping our brains and bodies functioning at a high level. If our body does not receive adequate, highly absorbable nutrition, our body can begin to send signals that some of its needs are not being met. Signals such as fatigue, hunger, irritability, inflammation, or feelings of sadness or panic may be signals that our body is not getting the proper amount of protein, fat, vitamins, or minerals.

Many health professionals focus solely on treating the symptoms of mental illnesses. This is usually done by prescribing one or more medications for the patient. While medications do have a place in alleviating acute symptoms, they should not be a substitute for exploring what is causing the symptoms in the first place. Perhaps more heartbreaking is that medication may only provide temporary relief or may completely fail to alleviate symptoms. In this case, an individual may feel that they will have to live a life plagued by anxiety, despair, and hopelessness.

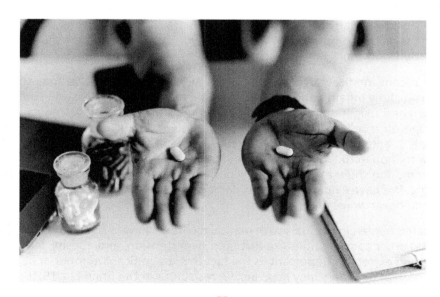

For many years, I lived with severe anxiety, episodes of depression, and constant, obsessive thoughts around food. I was convinced that these were simply the cards I was dealt, and I would have to deal with these struggles for the rest of my life.

During particularly difficult times in my life, I reached out for help and saw a therapist to discuss my anguish. I read books, studied papers, and talked to many nutrition professionals about the growing field of nutrition and mental health. I began to believe that a Mediterranean-type diet was the perfect solution to decrease my anxiety and bouts of depression.

It was my hypothesis that a diet rich in fruits and vegetables, due to the presence of antioxidants and fiber, low-to-moderate in protein, and low in added sugars was the perfect diet for depression. I believed that the brain loved colorful fruits and vegetables and adequate whole grains.

While I have always advocated for protein in the diet, I used to believe it should be a relatively small part of each meal. My small amount of low-fat protein was accompanied by a whole grain carbohydrate such as brown rice, and a large serving of vegetables, such as a massive salad. I dutifully followed this way of eating for many years, yet I experienced minimal relief related to my mental anguish. There were periods in my life where my depression became so severe, I experienced suicidal ideation and engaged in self-injury to the point of permanently scarring my wrists and arms. I am generally a happy, outgoing human. I did not understand why I could feel so low that I sought detrimental coping mechanisms to relieve my sadness.

I want you to think of the human brain as a supercomputer. It needs the right fuel at the right time or it will not work properly. If you input the wrong information into a computer, you are likely to have an error message flash at you. Most of us can relate to this frustration. If you keep inputting the wrong information the computer may freeze, lock you out, or completely shut down. The brain works in a similar fashion.

With recent medical advances, we are now able to measure various things that can show inflammation and oxidation in the brain. By measuring inflammation and oxidation, we can see when things are going awry and causing damage on a cellular level. It has been demonstrated that individuals with chronic mental disorders have elevated levels of lactate, free radicals, and inflammation in their brains. (10) Elevated levels of lactate, free radicals, and inflammation show that the brain is not working properly and damage is occurring. We have evidence that this damage is happening, but *why is happening and how can we prevent it?*

As stated earlier, individuals with mental disorders have a significantly higher risk for other comorbidities like diabetes, hypertension, and obesity. Interestingly, and extremely important, is the fact that a significant number of people with mental disorders may have insulin resistance in the brain (14,15,16)

For many years, it was thought that the brain did not need or utilize insulin. We now have very good data to show that *insulin is essential for the brain to function properly.* (17) What does it mean to have insulin resistance in the brain? Simply, if the brain is not able to utilize glucose from broken down carbohydrates, the brain cannot work right. Insulin resistance can show up in different areas of the brain and have different symptoms depending on the person. If a person's brain is not working correctly, this can lead to a depressed mood, suicidal ideation, hallucinations, an inability to determine fullness or hunger, and a constant, heightened sense of anxiety. (18)

How does an individual know they have insulin resistance in the brain? That's a great question. *It's possible to have insulin resistance in the brain even if you have normal blood glucose levels and no signs of diabetes.*

This means an individual with chronic, debilitating depression due to insulin resistance in the brain can go to their doctor, have a slew of medical tests run, and everything may come back in the normal range. This unfortunate reality has caused many individuals to leave a doctor's appointment with nothing more than a prescription for an antidepressant. If insulin resistance in the brain is the root cause, the individual with the mental illness is unlikely to have sustainable, long-term improvement in their mental health without addressing the foods they are eating.

If you or your loved one has experienced a dismissal of your anxiety, depression, or chronic mental distress due to normal lab values or have been told, "It's in your head," or "You need to think positively," I am here to apologize and offer an alternative idea. I hear you, and I believe you. This is not a story you are making up in your head, but it might very well be your brain's inability to break down and utilize certain foods.

There is a simple way to test if the foods you are eating are causing the mental illness or significantly exacerbating the symptoms. If you are feeling skeptical about this, I want to let you know I was right there with you. *How could something so simple have prevented decades of my suffering?* Every individual I have had the privilege to interview for my YouTube channel has shared the same gratitude. "I cannot believe how much better my anxiety became once I changed how I ate," was a common sentiment.

What if eating in this way was the ticket to beginning the healing process for many individuals with mental illness?

Studies show that reducing sugar and processed carbohydrates in your diet as well as engaging in exercise can have an impact on alleviating symptoms of depression. If you are eating the Standard American Diet, which is appropriately called the SAD diet, then eating more fruits and vegetables and decreasing desserts and soda may alleviate some depressive symptoms. In fact, a study looking at 23,245 measures in men and women between ages 39-83, found an adverse effect of higher sugar intake on mental health over a 5-year period. (19)

TOP NUTRIENTS FOR
BRAIN HEALTH

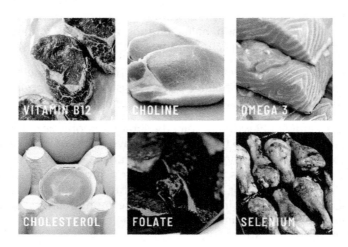

In my experience, many individuals struggling with mental illness are making an effort to follow a diet that includes whole grains, fruits, vegetables, and some low-fat protein. I noticed a trend at my last psychiatric hospital position where many patients were attempting to follow a vegetarian or vegan diet. Vegetarian diets are highly recommended by the Academy of Nutrition. Since many individuals dealing with mental illnesses are following the current nutrition recommendations set by the Academy of Nutrition, which includes fruits, vegetables, and lots of whole grains, why are we seeing little to no improvement in their symptoms?

When it comes to mental illnesses like major depressive disorder, anxiety disorders, bi-polar disorder, schizophrenia, and schizoaffective disorder, a bad diet *may not necessarily cause* insulin resistance in the brain.

Unlike type 2 diabetes, which is directly linked to diet, a poor diet ***does not always cause*** insulin resistance in the brain. Even a diet which is very high in processed carbohydrates and sugar, which can cause insulin resistance in the body, does not necessarily cause insulin resistance in the brain. A great way to understand this concept is to consider the medical condition epilepsy. Epilepsy is a neurological disorder marked by sudden recurrent episodes of sensory disturbance, loss of consciousness or convulsions, associated with abnormal electrical activity in the brain. Uncontrolled epilepsy results in seizures, falls, brain damage, and in severe cases, death. Since the 1920's it has been well established that epilepsy can be effectively treated with a ketogenic (very high fat, very low carbohydrate) diet. By utilizing ketones from fat instead of glucose from carbohydrates, many patients with epilepsy have been able to completely eliminate seizures without using medication. (20)

Toddlers and even infants can have epilepsy. Does an infant's bad diet cause the error of metabolism in the infant's brain? Of course not. That is absurd. No one was spiking their mother's breast milk or formula with sugar or high fructose corn syrup. The infant with epilepsy was simply born with an error in metabolism that prevents their brain from properly breaking down carbohydrates. This metabolic error generally goes undiagnosed until the infant has a seizure.

Once the parent knows their child has epilepsy, they have the option to place the child on a ketogenic diet. A ketogenic diet consists of 60-70% of calories coming from fat, 20-30% of calories coming from protein and 0-10% of calories coming from carbohydrates. *This way of eating allows the brain to utilize ketones instead of glucose.* A ketogenic diet has been deemed effective even in treating cases of drug resistant epilepsy. (20, 21, 22,23)

Dr. Chris Palmer states he has treated an individual with severe bipolar disorder and an individual with severe schizophrenia successfully with the ketogenic diet. Similarly, when individuals follow a diet with more protein and slightly less fat than a ketogenic diet, anxiety, depression, and mood disorders are remarkably improved as long as carbohydrate intake is kept low. By keeping fat intake high, protein intake moderate, and carbohydrate intake low, we see anecdotal evidence that an individual dealing with a mental illness who has insulin resistance in the brain can fuel their brain with ketones from fat instead of glucose from carbohydrates. This would, theoretically, allow their brain function properly.

I believe that the most powerful testimony you can share is your own. I decided to adopt a high-meat, high-fat, low-carbohydrate way of eating with the goal of alleviating my severe muscle pain. Within three weeks of adhering to this way of eating, my wife, who had known me then for eleven years, stated, "This is the best your anxiety has been since I've known you."

****

If we have clinical data to demonstrate that a lower carbohydrate, moderate protein, high-fat diet can potentially have a positive impact on improving mental health, why is this not presented as a treatment option for mental disorders? One factor preventing this approach is that we are an immediate gratification society. Giving someone a pill may provide immediate symptom relief, while a diet change could take a few weeks to months to fully manifest. Another potential barrier for implementing a low-carbohydrate, high-fat diet for this patient population, is the need to carefully monitor laboratory values and medications. Very low carbohydrate, high fat, moderate protein diets cause profound shifts in brain and body chemistry rather quickly. These changes are almost always positive and healthy, but they can have a major impact on medication levels, dosages, and side effects that require close medical supervision. This supervision is particularly crucial in the first month or two while metabolism adjusts to the new, low carbohydrate way of eating. As you can see, implementing this approach requires a medical provider who is familiar with low-carbohydrate diets, is willing to carefully monitor laboratory and medication levels, and who is open to feedback from the patient. I am grateful and encouraged by health care providers such as Dr. Palmer, who are committed to this type of collaborative low carbohydrate-based approach.

While I may sound like a broken record, our dietary guidelines are not designed for health. This will become even more apparent as you read through the chapter, "Where the F Did Our Dietary Guidelines Come From?" As I continued to listen to Dr. Chris Palmer speak, I could hear the anguish in his voice. He stated, "It's a political battle about money and power. The current dietary guidelines are the definition of insanity. We just keep doing the same damn thing over and over again with almost no changes and we somehow expect the American public is going to lose weight."

As a dietitian, I am often told by coworkers and leadership in my profession that the general public simply needs to follow the dietary guidelines to be healthy. I am told that *the guidelines are not the problem, lack of adherence to the guidelines* is the real issue. While I absolutely validate that there are people who live off cookies and fast food, data disagrees with this assertion.

Let's take a look at how Americans are eating. Data from 1970 to 2014 shows that we are actually consuming an estimated 9% more fruits and vegetables, 21% more wheat flour, and 114% more chicken than we did just a few decades ago. At the same time, were consuming less beef, less pork, and less eggs. Our consumption of animal fats such as butter is down, while our consumption of vegetable-based cooking oils such as canola, corn, soybean, and peanut oil is up. We now use over 200% more vegetable oils than we did in the 1970s. (24)

Although we are eating more "healthy" whole grains, plants, and less red meat and animal fats today than we did twenty years ago, we are continuing to get sicker and fatter.

In 1968, 3.18 million people were diagnosed with type 2 diabetes. As of 2015, the number has increased to 23.35 million. That is an increase of 734%. (25)

Currently, cardiovascular disease (CVD) is the number one killer in the United States. In 2006, health care spending and lost productivity from CVD exceeded $400 billion. (26) As you continue to read through this book and as we dive into our chapter on heart disease, you will learn how closely diabetes, mental illnesses, and heart disease are linked.

Another major issue with treating mental illness, is that many of the prescription drugs used to treat the symptoms of mental illnesses have been directly linked to an increased risk of weight gain, diabetes, and metabolic syndrome. Prescription drugs such as clozapine, olanzapine, risperidone, quetiapine, or haloperidol have been shown to either increase appetite or change metabolism, which can lead to weight gain. (27)

What are we serving in psychiatric hospitals across the nation?

You probably have an idea that the food served in mental institutions is not exactly filet mignon, but take a look at a menu approved by the Academy of Nutrition for our psychiatric population*:

Breakfast:

- Pancakes (2, white flour)
- Butter
- Imitation, high fructose corn syrup, maple syrup
- 4 ounces apple juice
- Banana
- 2 ounces of scrambled liquid eggs
- 2% milk

Breakfast

- Calories: 938
- Carbohydrates: 130
- **Sugar: 69 (17.25 teaspoons of sugar)**
- Protein: 28
- Fat: 34

Lunch

- 3-ounce roasted turkey with brown gravy
- Mashed potatoes with brown gravy
- Green beans
- Dinner roll
- Butter
- 4-ounce cup of diced peaches
- 2% milk
- Chocolate chip cookie

Lunch

- Calories: 893
- Carbohydrates: 110
- **Sugar: 46 (11.5 teaspoons of sugar)**
- Protein: 39
- Fat: 33

Dinner:

- Cheeseburger (3 oz patty, bun, 1-ounce cheddar cheese)
- Green salad with ranch
- 1 bag potato chips
- 4-ounce cranberry juice
- Sliced apples
- Chocolate ice cream

Dinner

- Calories: 820
- Carbohydrates: 93
- **Sugar: 53 (13.25 teaspoons of sugar)**
- Protein: 22
- Fat: 40

*Please note this does not include snacks provided. Snack examples:

- Peanut butter and jelly sandwich on white bread
- Hot chocolate (regular or sugar-free)
- Graham crackers or cereal bars

Daily Totals:
Calories: 2651
Carbohydrates: 333 (50%)
Sugar: 168 (42 teaspoons of sugar)
Protein: 89 (14%)
Fat: 107 (36%)

Percentage of Macronutrients Served to Patients:

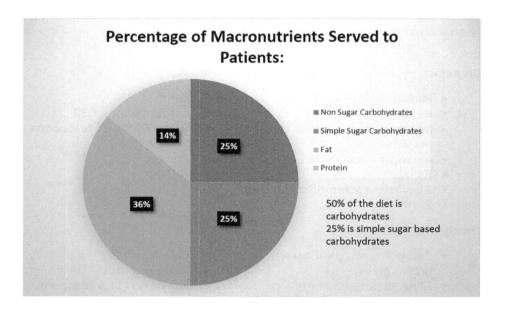

- Non Sugar Carbohydrates
- Simple Sugar Carbohydrates
- Fat
- Protein

50% of the diet is carbohydrates
25% is simple sugar based carbohydrates

Currently, we are feeding our patients suffering from mental illnesses *approximately 42 teaspoons of sugar a day.*

This is the equivalent of four 12-ounce cans of soda, every single day.

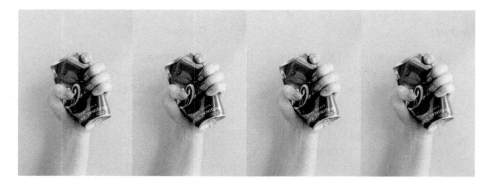

Just like consuming carbohydrates while diabetic is like setting your house on fire, consuming carbohydrates for a person with insulin resistance in the brain, is like setting your brain on fire.

I propose the radical solution of not setting your brain on fire. Interestingly, this is not a popular opinion in my profession. Many registered dietitians have been so indoctrinated with the false premise that humans require carbohydrates and sugar in moderation, that they cannot see the forest through the trees. They have lost the ability to think critically. To suggest that humans follow a high-fat, moderate protein, low-carbohydrate diet to return to health is blasphemy to many nutrition professionals.

Again, I am not anti-carbohydrate. Many people are able to metabolize and utilize *small* amounts of carbohydrates without any issues. On the same token, many people are not. To decide what approach will work for any individual, I recommend taking a step back and asking the question, "What is the number one goal for the individual?" For an individual with type 2 diabetes, an individual with a mental disease, or for an individual with a carbohydrate addiction, complete elimination of carbohydrates for a period of time may be helpful. Some people find long term elimination of carbohydrates necessary to heal and maintain health.

I have been fortunate to work with individuals with severe schizophrenia and bipolar disorder. The current nutrition guidelines do not allow me to advocate the high-fat, moderate protein, low-carb diet that I am describing in this book to these patients. I believe that **dietitians need to lead the charge** to work with doctors to help patients reduce or eliminate insulin regimens by reducing carbohydrates and increasing protein and fat. It is my belief that we could potentially see patients get off many psychiatric medications with this shift away from carbohydrates and towards fat and protein. Unfortunately, we are unlikely to see this in the clinical setting anytime soon.

As shown in the menu example above, it is standard to serve hospital patients more carbohydrates for breakfast (100-130 grams) than most people need over the course of an entire week. This many carbohydrates can be detrimental to brain health. Because it follows the current nutrition guidelines, carbohydrate and sugar intake is often not on the radar of health professionals as something that could cause or exacerbate mental illness.

If you or someone you care about is in the grips of a mental disorder, I encourage you to be open to fueling your body and brain in a way that is against the grain, but in line with human physiology. Having your brain function correctly will make every aspect of your life better.

Does someone need to completely eliminate all carbohydrates in order to heal?

I have had people tell me they would rather die than stop eating cookies or cake. I had a patient who had her leg amputated at the age of 48 due to complications for unmanaged diabetes. Less than 48 hours after her surgery, I watched her wheel herself down to the cafeteria for a donut because the hospital staff was restricting her carbohydrates intake.

Recall from the chapter on diabetes that the human body needs *zero carbohydrates* to function optimally, but it will die without eating adequate amounts of protein and fat. It is very difficult to overeat protein and fat in the absence of carbohydrates. The body releases various hormones and chemical messengers once protein and fat are consumed. In layman's terms, these messengers say, "Cool, keep going, I need these amino acids (protein) and fatty acids (fats)." Once you have consumed enough protein and fat, the body will send messages telling you, "I'm good, we can stop eating now."

This process of regulating appetite does not happen with carbohydrates. Many of my diabetic, mental illness, and heart disease patients have confessed to being able to eat an entire pint of ice cream, a full pizza, or a large cake in one sitting. Consuming a traditional breakfast of pancakes, fruit, and juice will provide an overwhelming number of calories, yet can leave you feeling hungry and exhausted a few hours later. Most people reading this will acknowledge that they have plowed through a bag of chips or a few rows of chocolate sandwich cookies at some point in their life. I most certainly have.

Not only does the body not self-regulate carbohydrate consumption, but it can also hijack neurotransmitters in the brain and trigger addiction-like behaviors. One study demonstrated that sugar, which is a simple carbohydrate, fit all the criteria of an addictive substance, causing behaviors such as bingeing, withdrawal, craving and cross-sensitization. (28) Many of the individuals I have interviewed for my YouTube channel described suffering with carbohydrate addiction to the point of having to completely abstain from carbohydrates in order to find freedom with food. Carbohydrates are not an essential nutrient, and I believe we have done a huge disservice prescribing them as the main portion of the human diet. As mentioned earlier, some people are able to tolerate small amounts of carbohydrates while some people are not.

You might think, *Okay, Michelle, I understand sugar is less than ideal. I understand refined carbohydrates, such as chips and cookies, are less than ideal. Are all carbohydrates potentially less than ideal for humans to consume?* All carbohydrate containing foods from white table sugar to apples are broken down into glucose or fructose in the body. All carbohydrates use similar pathways to be absorbed. A single banana or a mango can cause similar or even higher surges in blood sugar compared to a cookie or plate of pasta. *Even eating a whole food, high-carbohydrate diet can potentially exacerbate symptoms of mental health in susceptible individuals.* In my experience working in several psychiatric and acute care facilities, high-carbohydrate foods tend to make up most of the diet, and they often take the place of nutrient-dense, high protein foods.

For individuals with mental health illnesses, there appears to be potential benefits of carbohydrate restriction. When plants (carbohydrates) are eliminated for a set period of time, meat and fat provide most of the calories in the diet. This allows the brain to receive high quantities of amino acids, vitamins, minerals, and EPA and DHA.

If an individual is not ready or does not want to give up high-carbohydrate, high sugar foods such as soda, pasta, or cake, that's fine. If we have the mental capacity to do so, we should all be able to make our own choices when it comes to the foods we eat. That being said, I'd like to advocate that all health professionals provide information regarding a low-carbohydrate, high-fat diet and its potential benefits to individuals suffering with mental illnesses. This will allow the individual, or their guardian if they lack capacity, to understand the possible benefits and make an informed decision.

Are there other ways a high-fat, moderate protein, low-carbohydrate diet can heal the brain?

While we have discussed at length the connection between insulin resistance and mental health, are there other ways a high-fat, moderate protein, low-carbohydrate diet can maximize brain health? To answer this question, let's review information by Dr. Georgia Ede, psychiatrist and PHD.

In addition to errors in metabolism, Dr. Ede notes that providing adequate, highly absorbable nutrients to the brain and ensuring neurotransmitters are balanced are two essential components in maintaining mental health.

Dr. Ede agrees with Dr. Chris Palmer and shares his same exasperation by stating, "Whenever we see the dietary guidelines, we ignore the randomized controlled trials. Why? For brain health, they [controlled trials] all say that a low-carbohydrate, high-fat diet is better than a high-carbohydrate diet heavy in grains, fruits, and vegetables."

It seems to be ingrained in us from the time that we are small children that, "All fruits and vegetables are good for you." We are told, "Eat your vegetables." Interestingly, I have seen in my own practice, that people, especially as they age and are under stress, start to show signs of intolerance to certain plant foods.

I have heard patients say things such as, "Every time I eat bread, I feel awful," or, "I try to eat salads, but I'm massively bloated," as well as, "I feel anxious and hungry when I include lots of grains and vegetables in my diet." If our brain and bodies are designed to use these brightly colored foods, why do so many people have negative reactions to them? It is not uncommon for patients to tell me, "I've been good, I had a salad," and, "I'll be good and eat my broccoli." It seems that all of the plant kingdom is universally associated with eating well and contributing to health.

The human brain is mostly fat (approximately two thirds). The brain also contains protein and cholesterol. Cholesterol is so important that it exists in every cell membrane throughout the brain and body. The brain needs ketones or glucose, and it requires several vitamins and minerals to run the chemical reactions to function properly. Zinc, B6 and iron are essential in making neurotransmitters. The neurotransmitters that zinc, B6, and iron make are the same neurotransmitters that antidepressants are designed to boost. With such a high percentage of the United States population taking an antidepressant drug, does it not make sense that people would want to boost neurotransmitter activity naturally with food?

MORE THAN JUST
PROTEIN

BEEF
IRON
CREATINE
CLA
SELENIUM
VITAMIN B12

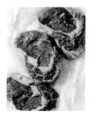

SALMON
OMEGA 3
POTASSIUM
SELENIUM
VITAMIN B6
VITAMIN D

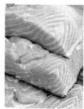

EGGS
BIOTIN
RIBOFLAVIN
FOLATE
VITAMIN B5
VITAMIN K2

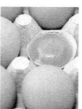

PORK
PHOSPHORUS
THIAMINE
RIBOFLAVIN
SELENIUM
VITAMIN B6

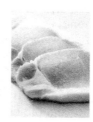

The quality of the macronutrients you eat will affect the micronutrient availability. This means that it will benefit you to eat high quality protein and fats in order to obtain forms of the micronutrients, such as vitamin B6, iron and zinc, that your brain can absorb and utilize.

Eating meat is the perfect way to ensure all the vitamins and minerals eaten are properly absorbed and utilized by the brain and body. Meat contains every nutrient in its proper form, and it contains no anti-nutrients, such as phytates, lectins, or oxalates, that will interfere with nutrient absorption.

Meat contains carnitine, which is a conditionally essential amino acid. The term conditionally essential means that the human body can make some carnitine, but often we aren't able to make it in the quantities that are required for optimal brain health. Carnitine is important for fluid and electrolyte balance in the brain. To make carnitine, we need lysine and methionine. These two amino acids are bioavailable in animal foods, and extremely hard to find in the plant kingdom.

Choline, which is found in meat and eggs, is an essential nutrient. It supports many bodily functions, including cellular growth, metabolism, and many other regulatory processes. A choline deficiency can result in poor concentration, difficulty with memory, severe mood swings and other cognitive impairments. High choline intake during gestational and early postnatal development has been shown to improve cognitive function in adulthood, prevents age-related memory decline, and protects the brain from the neuropathological changes associated with Alzheimer's disease (29).

Cholesterol continues to be a poorly misunderstood compound. While the brain only takes up 2% of the entire body weight, it contains 20% of the body's cholesterol. Many people have mistakenly followed a "low fat, low cholesterol diet" thinking this would be beneficial to the brain. We now know that cholesterol cannot cross the blood-brain barrier, meaning no matter how much or how little cholesterol we eat, the brain makes all of its own cholesterol.

Dr. Georgia Ede poses this question about cholesterol: "Why would the brain go out of its way to make a compound that could be potentially harmful to itself?" Recent articles have gone on to say that cholesterol may indeed be really good for brain health. In fact, higher cholesterol as we age may lead to better brain health. One particular study of older people found that those aged 85–94 who had a total cholesterol level higher than they had in midlife had a lower risk of marked cognitive decline. (30)

Neurotransmitters and the Brain:

When the word "neurotransmitter" comes up, most people think of serotonin and dopamine. Serotonin is important in regulating neurological processes such as mood and social behavior, appetite and digestion, sleep, memory, and sexual desire and function. In addition, serotonin regulates numerous biological processes including cardiovascular function, bowel motility, and bladder control. (31)

Dopamine is a neurotransmitter that plays a part in motor control, motivation, reward/pleasure, and cognitive function. (32)

Two of the most prevalent neurotransmitters in the brain, glutamate and gamma-aminobutyric acid (or GABA) are less known. Understanding these neurotransmitters is essential when it comes to mental illness and overall brain health. We know that imbalances in dopamine, glutamine, or GABA can contribute to mental disorders, but what is causing these imbalances? Let's take a look at the kynurenine pathway (KPW).

Let's say a person eats eggs or a large chicken thigh, both of which are rich sources of tryptophan. Some of this tryptophan will be used to make serotonin to regulate mood. Some of the tryptophan will enter the KPW. Once it enters this pathway, the specific reactions occur to ensure that glutamate activity is balanced. Some activity with be activated, while some will be inhibited.

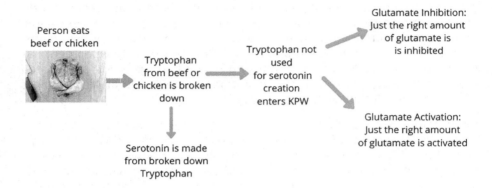

What happens if we have too much glutamate in the brain? Excessive glutamate over time can cause brain damage. It also decreases a very important neurotrophic factor, brain-derived neurotrophic factor, or BDNF.

BDNF is responsible for helping the human brain cope with stress. Stress is a normal part of life. Being able to cope, process, and move on from the many stressors a person will face in life is an essential part of being a functioning, competent person. We are seeing a spike in individuals not being able to cope with even normal amounts of stress. Could this be tied to the brain being flooded with glutamate?

When you eat highly processed carbohydrates, sugar, or seed oils, you create oxidation and inflammation. Tryptophan is no longer able to perform its functions. In this case, you get what is called "tryptophan steal." Instead of making serotonin, tryptophan is shuttled towards glutamate activation. *This can create up to 100 times more glutamate than the brain needs to function optimally.* At the same time the brain is being flooded with glutamate, you get an increase in dopamine signaling, which causes pleasurable feelings. This is one of the many reasons eating highly processed foods is so dangerous. While damaging the body and brain, it actually sends messages to your brain (via dopamine) saying, "This is great, I feel happy and calm."

Immediately after eating a high-carbohydrate or high sugar meal, most of us feel a sense of pleasure, calm, or peace. *Once the dopamine high from the carbohydrates wears off, some individuals come down hard and can experience extreme sadness or become emotionally distraught.* It is not uncommon to have strong feelings of guilt, anxiety, or difficulty coping with basic life stressors for several hours after a highly refined carbohydrate-filled meal. *Keep in mind that food manufacturers understand and use this to their advantage.* They are counting on their consumers to repeat the cycle, seeking the high that sugar and carbohydrates provide. The fact that this is detrimental to an individual's mental health is not their concern. **To health professionals, especially dietitians, I believe it should be.**

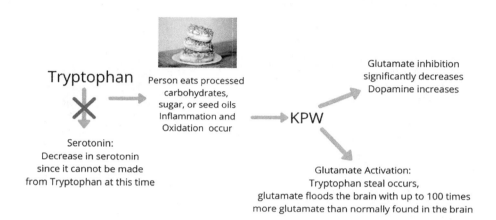

Tryptophan

Person eats processed carbohydrates, sugar, or seed oils Inflammation and Oxidation occur

Serotonin: Decrease in serotonin since it cannot be made from Tryptophan at this time

KPW

Glutamate inhibition significantly decreases Dopamine increases

Glutamate Activation: Tryptophan steal occurs, glutamate floods the brain with up to 100 times more glutamate than normally found in the brain

So far, we have discussed how mental disorders are potentially linked to errors in metabolism, nutrient deficiencies, and imbalances of neurotransmitters. All of these have the potential to be reversed or significantly improved with a low-carbohydrate, high-fat, moderate protein (meat) diet. In later chapters, we will review the specifics of why plant foods might not be the best answer for human health, and I will answer your questions about fiber, antioxidants, and concerns for LDL and total cholesterol. Now, it's time to move onto a chapter that I found challenging, as well as liberating, to write. Let's discuss eating disorders.

Trudy Miller

Email: CarnivoreCoachTrudy@gmail.com
Facebook: Trudy Miller
Instagram: trudylmiller

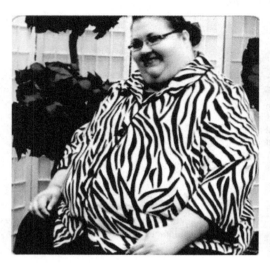 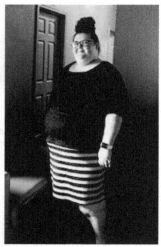

Never in my wildest nightmares could I ever have imagined that I would one day weigh nearly 500 pounds! I was a preemie, weighing only 3lbs, 13oz at birth. I was a tiny child, weighing much less than other kids my age. It was not until my teen years that weight became a problem for me. In my mid-teens, I was a little overweight compared to my friends, but I wasn't what you would call "fat" by any means. By the time I was 18, I weighed 198 pounds!

I was told that I'd never find a man because I was overweight, so I didn't try. Then, someone came through selling "all-natural herbal weight loss miracle pills." I started taking them and drinking weight loss shakes. I ended up taking nearly 3 times the recommended doses per day. They were like speed! And yes, they did make me lose weight! Within 4 months, I'd lost 83 lbs., but the pills had caused damage to my heart. I couldn't even drink caffeine without my heart racing out of control. But hey, I was down to 115 pounds, so it worked! *ugh*

The thing about any diet (including pills) is that you tend to gain once you go off the diet. Well, once I stopped taking the pills and drinking the weight loss shakes, and I was actually eating food, I gained about 25 lbs. A year later, I was married. I weighed around 140, which wasn't horrible, and no one even believed I weighed that much.

Shortly after marriage, we were expecting our first baby. I gained weight rather quickly, wearing maternity clothes just 10 weeks into my pregnancy. I continued to gain rapidly, all the while eating sensibly with only a little splurging. My only craving was french fries from our local fast-food place in town. They were the best fries ever!

Just 3 weeks before my baby was due, I had to have an emergency C-section due to out-of-control blood pressure. It was nearly stroke level (210/115), and they were afraid the baby and I would both stroke out if they didn't take her early. I weighed 236 when she was born, meaning I'd gained 94 lbs. during my pregnancy. It was unbelievable! After the baby was born, my health continued to decline. My nerves got so bad that I had trouble taking care of myself, much less a husband and our newborn daughter who was born with spina bifida. I asked my parents to take her until the day came that I was mentally and physically capable of caring for her.

Having to give up custody of our daughter did not seem to help my nerve situation, but it did make me feel better knowing that I did what was best for the baby who was 3 months old when we finally had to give her up. It was the hardest thing I've ever had to do in my entire life!

Over the next few years, I suffered severe postpartum depression symptoms. Then I ended up on blood pressure medication and meds for hypothyroidism. The doctor said my thyroid tests came back negative, but she couldn't find another reason for my constant weight gain, so she put me on a thyroid pill. No joke!

I developed asthma after getting pneumonia, and I ended up with an inhaler. I was also on a fluid pill and 2 different meds for my nerves, neither of which were helping at all, so I stopped taking them. During all this time, I continued to gain weight without rhyme or reason. I developed severe acid reflux, severe anxiety, severe sleep apnea (which caused me to stop driving), headaches, migraines, chronic sinusitis, and severe seasonal allergies. I was so big that we stopped going to shopping malls. I had to get dropped off at restaurant doors and at the doors of church or any store because I couldn't walk far.

In July 2011, things went from bad to worse! It was the week of my 31st birthday, and I was feeling even more awful than usual. I couldn't eat, had no appetite, and could only drink water and eat popsicles. I just felt so bad. It didn't help that I then weighed nearly 500 lbs.!

I drank a case of water, and my vision got blurry so my husband decided to rush me to the ER. They checked my glucose level and it was too high to register so they had to take blood and send it to the lab. My sugar was over 600, and my A1C was 11. The doctor came in and said "So you know you're a diabetic now". I was in ICU for the next couple days, then they moved me to a regular room where they began to educate me on type 2 diabetes, and how to manage it.

I was told to eat no more than 45g carbs per meal, and to watch for hidden sugars in prepackaged foods and salad dressings. The dietitian told me I could have some birthday cake if we were celebrating, or something sweet every once in a while, as long as I didn't overdo it. That was pretty much all the education I got. I immediately quit sugar, which I thought would be really difficult. I grew up in the Deep South where you drank sweet tea from sunup to sundown, and had bread and rice, potatoes, or pasta at every meal. I was pleasantly surprised that I didn't miss the sugar, though I did miss potatoes.

I was 31, I'd lost my 20's to morbid obesity and extremely poor health, and I was determined to be a "good diabetic" and do everything I was told! I watched my carbs, took my Glucotrol and metformin, and tried to do every-thing I could. Within 15 months or so I'd lost 100 pounds! I maintained that weight loss for the next few years, not losing but not gaining either so I was okay with that.

Only July 28, 2019, I woke up that morning and said, "I'm starting Keto!" With-in a month I was off diabetes meds and cholesterol meds. I also no longer needed my walking cane! Within 5 months of starting Keto, I'd lost 60 lbs. I felt amazing! But I was still on meds for anxiety, high blood pressure, acid reflux, and seasonal allergies, and I wanted to eliminate them also.

I came across some Carnivore (high-meat, no plants) people while research-ing Keto, and I was like, "No way will I ever give up my veggies!" It was hard enough to give up fruit when I went Keto. I just couldn't imagine a diet where you ate no plants at all. At Christmas of 2019 I decided to try Carnivore for 30 days. I wanted to see if it would help the inflammation I was experiencing. I currently weigh 320, but that's a long way from where I started at nearly 500 pounds!

I'm currently studying to be a Carnivore coach. I also hope to start doing some motivational speaking maybe next year. My dream is to help others who feel hopeless, helpless, and can't see their life being any different. I'm so grateful to have found the keto/carnivore way of eating! It's not a diet, it's a way of life! I will never go back to putting sugar and junk into my body. I can hardly wait to see what the future holds!

Heather Le Gaux

Instagram: https://www.instagram.com/heathernicoleco/
Website: https://www.heathernicole.co/
You Tube: https://www.youtube.com/c/HeatherLeGaux

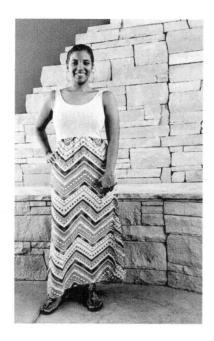

I found out about the Carnivore way of eating when I was 39. A friend of mine tried it, and I was completely intrigued. I did some research and watched endless YouTube videos of people's experiences on a carnivore diet and quickly jumped in. I did not take baby steps. I did not slowly reduce my carbs. I went cold turkey.

I have spent most of my adult life trying to find the perfect way of eating for me. Some of the diets I tried in the past were raw vegan, low-fat, high-carb vegan, The Perfect Health Diet, The Bulletproof Diet, The Paleo Diet, and The Ketogenic Diet. My main struggles were fatigue and hair loss. Other issues I'd been looking to resolve included morning grogginess, brain fog, food cravings, mild depression/anxiety and tooth sensitivity. Some of the diets I mentioned did help with these things, but none seemed to be the perfect fit for me for one reason or another.

When I started the carnivore diet, I experienced the mental health benefits almost immediately; I would say it was less than 10 days. I felt incredibly calm and my ability to handle stress went up. I slept better and began to think very clearly. My ability to focus for long periods improved a lot. I lost 2 dress sizes – I went from a size 12 to a size 8. This was not immediate but happened within 3 months. I noticed my hair loss slowed to the point where I barely lost any hair at all. After the first 6 weeks, my energy skyrocketed. My teeth were no longer sensitive either. All in all, everything I was looking to resolve had been resolved. Also, this diet is so easy to implement once you wrap your head around it. I only spend a fraction of the time that I was used to preparing food and even grocery shopping is quick and easy. The unexpected benefit of getting so much of my precious time back has been a true delight.

It has now been two years and I still eat a whole food meat-based diet. I do not incorporate any plant foods except coffee. I have all the energy I need to do everything I set out to do each day. I currently keep my hair short, but it is full and much thicker than it used to be. I feel great every day and would not trade it for the world.

Chapter 3

Eating Disorders: Silently Destroying the Soul

Here I Am Again

Here I am again; I know this feeling so well

This emptiness, this powerlessness, this emotional hell

In times like this, I know exactly what I need to do,

I should surrender to recovery, and to my program be true.

But thinking about changing my self-destructive patterns and behaviors

Brings fear and anxiety; and from my disorder I choose NOT to waiver

And before I can begin to think anything else; oh it happens so fast

Here I am AGAIN doing the same behaviors, shamefully repeating the past

I know I want to change but I have no idea how I will do it

I can't face myself; I don't have the strength to fight and pull through it

I am standing in the moment; I know what I need to do

I have a meal plan to follow, a plan to surrender to

And I have things I can do when I don't want to eat,

A journal to write in or a friend I can call; she's always willing to meet

Yet I block everyone out, and keep my pain to myself,

I am a prisoner to my desperations; terrified to ask for help

I walk to the bathroom to splash cold water on my face

I glance in the mirror; all I see is a total disgrace

I put my hand on the mirror my eyes filled with tears

This person staring back at me is consumed with self-loathing and is completely defeated by their fears

When I stare at this person, I cry out loud, "WHO IS THIS?"

This person terrified of food and of weight, and with scars up and down their wrists

And what would happen if I decided to face my fears?

And put behind the lying, the deceit, and forget my wasted years

But when I think about facing my fears and trying to eat

My thoughts are flooded with visions of my past defeats

Anger consumes me, I pound my fist into the wall

WHO is this monster I see? I don't know this person at all!

I have been living a life fueled by my twisted sense of control

I am broken beyond repair; I will never again be made whole

I don't want anyone to worry, it's not like I am dying

I been to hospitals twice, and honestly, I'm tired of trying

What I would give for just 10 seconds of-peace

To look into this mirror and have my anxieties release

And maybe just for an instant I could see what others do

Maybe that would allow me to believe what they are saying is true

Everyone is telling me I look pale, sick, and terribly thin,

I am in a battle with myself; and it's a battle I can't win

What I wouldn't give to look into my reflection and see

A strong, independent young woman; the person I used to dream I could be

My truth is much different than theirs, my disorder defines me

It controls everything I do, and it constantly reminds me

All I have to do to feel good about myself is to continue to live in it

I don't have the strength to fight it, and more often than not, I lie and defend it

Yet in all of this, one fact continues to remain

I will always see myself as worthless and fat; this truth will never change

I turn away from the mirror and close my eyes

Its moments like this that make me want to die

How can anyone be so selfish, so stubborn, so caught up in their self

That they would rather starve themselves to death than honestly seek help?

I hate myself and the pain I have caused my family

I can't help but wonder if they would be better off without me.

Everyone tells me, "Recovery is a choice you have to make"

They don't know I am a failure, a hopeless cause, and a fake

And I'm sitting here wondering how much longer I can keep this up

I don't know how to change, I'll starve myself until my time is up

Sometimes I wonder if I'll ever be able to stop

I starve myself, binge, purge, and exercise until I drop

And I am feeling so tired so incredibly down

My life feels meaningless, and I doubt it will ever turn around

I had something to eat within the last hour

When I allow myself to have food, I lose all sense of control and of power

And I tell myself that this will be it for the day, this will be the last time

After this I am going to go lie down and try to forget the thoughts running through my mind

After I purge I'll go rest in my sorrows

Maybe I'll find some courage and ask for help tomorrow

Some people say, that if I purge too much I could die

But that's just something they make up, that's surely a lie...

Written in Memory of Mary* who passed away from bulimia at the age of 15

This may be a difficult chapter to read as it challenges the current dogma and many of the recommendations around eating disorder treatment, recovery, and relapse prevention. I encourage you to approach this chapter with an open mind. *If you are currently in recovery, make sure you have adequate support before making any changes to your current treatment regimen.* There are several resources throughout this book to help you get started if you choose to do so.

In this chapter, we will be diving into the current dietary recommendations for individuals with eating disorders. We will break down what happens in the body and brain when an individual follows the current Academy of Nutrition guidelines, and we will discuss an alternative way of eating. We will explore if this way of eating may be a better, long term option for an individual in recovery. Then, we will review therapeutic modalities and discuss their essential role in recovery. I'll share my hypothesis regarding a combination of a specific way of eating combined with therapeutic modalities and how this combination can facilitate healing and rewiring of the brain while rebuilding the muscle tissues throughout the body. Interestingly, this alternative approach may be helpful in preventing relapse.

I have often thought I would write an entire book about what it is like to live bound by the chains of an eating disorder. In the past, whenever I began to write about my experience, I became paralyzed with fear. How could the written word capture the depths of the physical and mental suffering I personally experienced? How could I express the pain, anguish, and complete despair that my loved ones felt seeing their daughter, sister, friend, and wife, slowly starve themselves, engage in self-injury, and lie about it? What is it like for a mother to hear that their child has a 10% chance of survival? Would I seem selfish to admit I felt genuine gratitude and relief instead of shame and fear when I heard the doctor tell my parents that I "likely wouldn't survive"? Death became a welcome alternative to living with a disorder that was destroying my body and occupying every waking moment of my thoughts. *Finally.* I remember thinking all those years ago. *It's almost over.*

Throughout my entire adolescence and into adulthood, I lived what I thought was to be my fate of perpetual, obsessive, eating disordered thoughts. I was no longer in danger of dying from the side effects of starvation or undereating, but I was constantly analyzing, judging, overthinking, and reanalyzing every morsel of food I put into my mouth. Did I eat the right amount of protein, fat, and carbohydrate? Did my stomach hurt? Did I eat too much? Did I eat too little? I was anxious, depressed, and I isolated frequently. In times of extreme stress, I found refuge in new, unhealthy coping mechanisms. While doing research for this book, I discovered it is not unusual for individuals with eating disorders to trade one unhealthy coping mechanism for another. They may cease to overexercise or consciously undereat, only to become addicted to unhealthy relationships, alcohol, or drugs. (1) *If you've fallen into this category, know that you're not alone.*

I have been told by more than one professional and several individuals in recovery from various eating disorders that, "You never fully recover." This phrase has a different meaning depending on who you talk to. The consensus is that once you have an eating disorder you can heal your physical body, but it will always be in your thoughts, to some degree. You have the choice whether to act on the impulses to binge, purge, compulsively exercise, or starve yourself, but the painful, obsessive thoughts and feelings of self-hatred will likely be a source of reoccurring trauma throughout your life.

What exactly causes one to develop an eating disorder or eating disordered tendencies? Eating disorders tend to develop from a perfect storm of genetic and environmental factors. Risk factors found to precede an eating disorder include sex, ethnicity, early childhood eating and gastrointestinal problems, elevated weight and shape concern, negative self-evaluation, sexual abuse and other traumas. (2) Prospective studies indicate an individual may be at risk if they perceive a pressure to be thin, they idealize the idea of thinness, or have body dissatisfaction. (3). Unfortunately, this line of thinking describes many preteens and teenagers in America. An article published in *Time Magazine* in 2019 stated, "According to the CDC, from 2013 to 2016, almost 38% of American adolescents ages 16 to 19 said they had tried to lose weight during the past year." That is an increase from 25% of adolescents who said the same thing a decade ago, according to previous research. Genetics certainly play a role as a predisposing factor to eating disorders. (4,5) To what degree, nature versus nurture, we do not know.

When the term "eating disorder" comes up, many people imagine an emaciated white female. In reality, eating disorders impact all ages, genders, races and ethnic groups. (6,7) At least 30 million people in the United States suffer from eating disorders, and the number is estimated to be over 70 million people worldwide. Men, who account for 10% of eating disorders, have an immense stigma to overcome. (8) Over 16% of transgender college students report having an eating disorder. (9) While eating disorders tend to start in early adolescence, 13% of women over the age of 50 engage in eating disorder behaviors. (10)

There are several types of eating disorders. Below, the dynamics and current treatment regimens for anorexia, bulimia, binge eating disorder, and orthorexia will be discussed.

> Anorexia has one of the highest mortality rates of any mental illness. Approximately 1 in 10 cases of anorexia ends in death.

Anorexia is an eating disorder characterized by either weight loss, or lack of appropriate weight gain in children, and difficulty maintaining an appropriate body weight for height, age, and stature. Many individuals with anorexia have a distorted body image and see themselves as significantly larger and heavier than they are. People with anorexia tend to restrict food and compulsively count calories, as well as track, judge, and analyze the foods they eat. According to the Academy of Nutrition, the current role of the dietitian in an eating disorder treatment protocol is "to work as part of a multidisciplinary team, to challenge distorted and irrational thinking about food and weight, and to explore feelings related to hunger, fullness, metabolism, and body image." (11) While this sounds great in theory, what does this actually mean in practice? The dietitian will design a meal plan using our current nutrition guidelines. This involves having the patient eat several high-calorie, high-carbohydrate meals and snacks.

Below is an example of a 3,000-calorie sample weight gain meal plan. This is based on the exchange system that divides foods into categories including starch, fat, meat, milk, fruit, and vegetable. This system assumes that all foods groups are necessary regardless of disease state (physical or mental) or issues with metabolism such as diabetes. Analyzing and overanalyzing various food group exchanges can become a new, unhealthy obsession for individuals with eating disorders.

Breakfast: 2 Starch, 1 Fat, 2 Meat, 1 Milk, 2 Fruit

- 2 4-inch pancakes (2 starch exchanges) with 1 tsp. butter (1 fat exchange)
- 2 scrambled eggs (2 meat exchanges)
- 8 ounces of while milk (1 milk exchange)
- 4 oz of orange juice & 1/2 a banana (2 fruit exchanges)

Lunch: 2 Starch, 2 Vegetable, 3 Meat, 2 Fat, 1 Milk

- Grilled cheese sandwich: 2 slices of whole wheat bread (2 starch exchanges), 2 tsp margarine (2 fat exchanges), 3 slices of cheddar cheese (3 meat exchanges)
- Tomato soup: 1 cup tomato soup condensed (2 vegetable exchanges) made with 1 cup whole milk (1 milk exchange)

Dinner: 4 Starch, 3 Meat, 3 Fat, 2 Vegetable, 1 Fruit

- 1 cup cooked whole wheat pasta (2 starch exchanges)
- 2 pieces garlic toast (2 starch exchanges) + 2 tsp margarine (2 fat exchanges)
- 3 oz of ground turkey (3 meat exchanges) browned in 1 tsp olive oil (1 fat exchange)
- ½ cup tomato sauce with ½ cup cooked broccoli (2 vegetable exchanges)
- 1 orange (1 fruit exchange)

Snack #1: 2 Starch, 1 Milk

- 1 large blueberry muffin (2 starch exchanges 1 fat exchange)
- 1 cup whole milk (1 milk exchange)

Snack #2: 1 Fruit, 1 Milk

- 1 orange (1 fruit exchange)
- 1 cup whole milk, blueberry yogurt (1 milk exchange)

Snack #3: 1 Meat, 2 Starch, 1 Vegetable, 1 Fat

- 1 tbsp peanut butter (1 meat exchange)
- 2 sourdough bread slices (2 starch exchanges)
- 1 cup raw celery (1 vegetable exchange), 1 oz hummus (1 fat exchange)

Is this the best way to refeed a person whose body and brain is damaged and inflamed from prolonged starvation and abuse? Will this meal plan provide adequate fat, saturated fat, high quality protein, highly absorbable vitamins and minerals? Make no mistake, this way of eating will lead to weight restoration. The person in recovery will inevitably put on muscle and fat mass eating this way. If the first principal of medicine is to cause no harm, are we sure that this way of eating will not do just that?

I'd like to ask an uncomfortable question, challenging the current dogma.

Is this the *best way of eating* to set up an individual with anorexia for long term recovery? Does this way of eating allow for mood stabilization and help the brain heal? Could this way of eating increase inflammation and exacerbate anxiety?

Eating this many carbohydrates, many of which are processed and dense in sugar, can set the individual up for a pretty rough blood sugar roller coaster ride. See chart below:

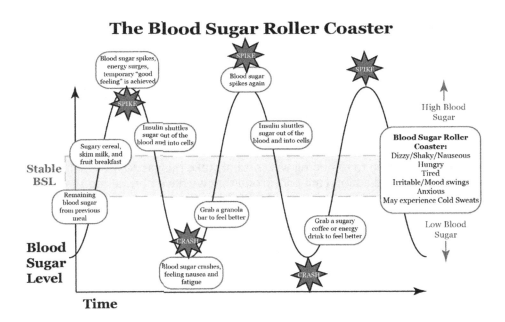

The Blood Sugar Roller Coaster

Even though current nutrition recommendations will design meals with some protein and fat, my experience has shown me that these meals tend to be woefully inadequate in *high quality* fats and *bioavailable*, meaning the body can use it, proteins.

The digestive system of a person with anorexia tends to be inflamed and motility is slow due to underfeeding. Feeding this person things like oats, vegetables, fruit, and chocolate milk provides starch, fiber, and a significant amount of sugar. Adding sugar and fiber to a damaged gastrointestinal tract may cause unpleasant side effects such abdominal pain, nausea, bloating, and gas. High fiber items may cause the individual to feel like they have a brick sitting in their stomach. Constipation, diarrhea or a combination of the two might follow. Assisting the individual with anorexia in trading a restriction-based way of eating for the Standard American Diet may initially save the individuals life by providing calories. Unfortunately, it may also set them up for years of generalized anxiety, depression, or other health issues such as chronic nausea, constipation, diverticulitis, small bowel obstruction, and other gastrointestinal difficulties. If you have been in recovery and have been fed this type of meal plan, you have likely experienced some, or perhaps many, of the symptoms referenced. Throughout my recovery I personally experienced many of these symptoms.

If you have struggled mightily with anxiety and gastrointestinal distress, know that there is nothing fundamentally wrong with you. There is a flaw in the system, and I think we can do much better.

As I was reviewing meal plans for individuals with anorexia, I came across a dietitian's blog. This particular dietitian worked specifically with individuals struggling with eating disorders. In her blog, she wrote in detail about how weight restoration meal plans may cause gastrointestinal issues, such as severe bloating, constipation, diarrhea, headaches, night sweats, low blood sugar, and increased anxiety. She went on to say that all of these things are "common," when the gastrointestinal tract is getting used to processing a greater volume of food. Yes, if you are following the Academy of Nutrition recommendations, these symptoms are common. While transitioning from extreme starvation to refeeding will certainly take the gastrointestinal system time to adjust and adapt, I am concerned that we have normalized the avoidable suffering that the Academy of Nutrition dietary approach may cause. The individual with an eating disorder will be told that it "just takes time," for their system to adapt, while the excessive amount of carbohydrates and sugar can wreak havoc on the brain and body. At this point, the individual suffering will likely be prescribed a cocktail of anti-anxiety, anti-depressant, and anti-nausea prescription medications.

It seems to make more sense to refeed individuals suffering with anorexia in a way of eating that aligns with human physiology. This same way of eating keeps inflammation low and keeps blood sugar and hormone levels stable. Simply keeping blood sugar and hormones stable can have a profound impact on minimizing anxiety. Eating in a way that aligns with human physiology actually *prevents* bloating, abdominal pain, and allows for normal, easy bowel movements. No long-term medication required. We will continue to discuss this later in the chapter, but now let's move on and address bulimia.

Bulimia is defined by recurrent episodes of binge eating followed by purging. A binge eating episode is defined as eating a large amount of food, which is generally high in calories, in a short period of time. A binge can consist of almost any food item, and it often comes down to what is available in terms of food and finance. Binge eating tends to occur in secrecy and is characterized by rapid, frenzied consumption. After a binge, the individual with bulimia will engage in a purging behavior. In the case of bulimia, a purge is defined as a behavior to remove the body of food items in an attempt to avoid weight gain. 70-80% of individuals suffering with bulimia will purge by self-induced vomiting. (12) Other individuals may choose to take laxatives, exercise excessively, or fast for prolonged periods of time. (12) A person with bulimia as well as binge eating disorder, which is detailed below, often has turned to food for comfort and to deal with difficult emotions and trauma. The recurrent binge-and-purge cycles of bulimia can affect several major organ systems and can lead to electrolyte and chemical imbalances in the body.

I wrote the poem featured at the beginning of this chapter shortly after I suffered the stress fracture that ended my college running career. At the time, I was 18. I was struggling with my own demons, and I found solace in honoring a friend I met during my time in inpatient eating disorder treatment years prior. I met Mary* at Remuda Ranch, and she told me I was, "one of the ones that would make it." At the time, I had no idea why she was so adamant I would recover. She was equally as adamant that she was "too far gone," and probably would not live to be 20. Like many individuals with eating disorders, she was witty, intelligent, stubborn, and had profoundly low self-esteem combined with crippling anxiety. At the age of 15, she suffered a heart attack during a bulimic episode of purging. She didn't survive.

Binge eating disorder is the most common eating disorder in the United States, affecting an estimated 2.3 million people. (13) Binge eating disorder is a serious, life-threatening disorder characterized by recurrent episodes of eating large quantities of food, often, in a short period of time. Individuals with binge eating disorder will feel a loss of control during the binge, and they often experience extreme, overwhelming feelings of shame, guilt, and self-hatred afterwards. Unlike individuals with bulimia, individuals with binge eating disorder do not engage in unhealthy compensatory measures such as self-induced vomiting or excessive exercise. The dietitian working with an individual with bulimia and binge eating disorder will use the same high-carbohydrate, highly processed "food" guidelines as they did for the individual with anorexia.

While I can see a *possible rationale* for an initial prescription of a carbohydrate heavy diet to ensure rapid weight gain for an individual with anorexia whose weight is dangerously low, I am at a loss to rationalize this way of eating for individuals suffering with bulimia or binge eating disorder. The only rationale is that these outdated nutrition guidelines continue to be the "standard" of practice by the Academy of Nutrition. In my professional experience, these guidelines rarely equal long-term physical or mental health. They do continue to make a lot of money for the processed food and pharmaceutical industry. Recall that some processed food companies funnel thousands of dollars to the Academy of Nutrition through sponsorship. We will go into great detail about this potential conflict of interest in our chapter about the origins of the nutrition guidelines. The current nutrition guidelines have the potential to keep individuals attempting to recover constantly relapsing. If you are currently suffering from an eating disorder and have experienced tremendous guilt and shame after a relapse, I hope my story and experience offer you encouragement and a belief in true recovery. There is a different way to eat. *You have an alternative option to explore when it comes to providing your body with nourishment.*

As stated above, carbohydrate heavy nutrition guidelines often lead to blood sugar spikes and crashes. When blood sugar crashes, hormones are released to signal that it is time to eat. Although a person eating a carbohydrate heavy diet is often lacking in protein and essential vitamins and minerals, this does not mean the person *physically needs calories.* I have seen an individual eat a meal containing over 1,000 calories and over 200 grams of carbohydrates. This meal was so carbohydrate heavy, it contained several servings of pasta, a roll, salad, and a large glass of sweet tea and a dessert, that the pancreas overproduced insulin. This overproduction of insulin, which is designed to shuttle the carbohydrates out of the blood stream, caused their blood sugar level to go too low. This crash causes the body to think it needs food even though significant calories were consumed. This individual's body was telling them to "eat again, blood sugar is low," less than two hours after consuming the high-carbohydrate meal. This way of eating is overriding the body's built in hormonal signals to regulate true hunger and fullness.

If you are trying to gain weight to prevent mortality, a high-carbohydrate, high-sugar way of eating could be a short-term, positive thing for you. For most humans and for individuals struggling with bulimia or binge eating disorder, experiencing blood sugar spikes, crashes, and subsequent hunger is not only confusing, it can set them up to engage in harmful behaviors and stunt recovery.

Eating a very high calorie, high carbohydrate diet has demonstrated via multiple clinical trials that it can cause blood sugar spikes, crashes, and weight gain. (14,15,16,17) Should we encourage individuals to eat a "balanced, whole grain heavy diet" even if it could set them up to feel hungry, dizzy, and fatigued hours after eating? We have statistical data that shows women with anorexia, bulimia, and binge eating disorder have increased rates of major depression relative to the general population. (4,5) Might this processed carbohydrate heavy, sugar-dense way of eating be a contributing factor?

As nutrition professionals, might it be helpful to teach the option of eating in a way that not only provides highly satiating, nutritious foods but also keeps blood sugar and hormone levels in their optimal range? For many individuals, following this way of eating has allowed them to make peace with food over time. In my personal and clinical experience, this way of eating has the potential to provide the proper nutrition for the brain to process trauma and rewire. If someone is making the effort to process their trauma and work through their issues, would their recovery journey *be helped, not hindered* by a diet that supports their brain function, metabolic rate, and aligns with human physiology? I have found it fascinating that merely suggesting a way of eating that differs from our current nutrition guidelines is often met with objection and disapproval.

Let's move on and discuss the dynamics of orthorexia. Orthorexia is an eating disorder that is not formally recognized by the Diagnostic and Statistical Manual, but awareness of this disorder continues to rise. The term "orthorexia" was coined in 1998, and it is defined as an obsession with healthful eating. Since you are currently reading this, it is safe to say you appreciate the importance of the type of food you are putting into your body and how it impacts your health. While adjusting the foods you eat has the potential to heal your brain and body, obsessing about the minutia to the point that it paralyses your ability to function is certainly not healthy!

A person with orthorexia often cuts out any food or food group they deem to be "unhealthy" including meat, eggs, butter, and anything with saturated fat. Unfortunately, a person with orthorexia may undergo treatment where they are taught that "all foods can fit" and "all things in moderation." **While this message may initially feel liberating and empowering, it's my experience that in the long term, it exacerbates the problem.** Substituting an orthorexic view of health for the Standard American Diet (SAD) is the equivalent of trading one unhealthy way of thinking about and eating food for an equally unhealthy way of thinking about and eating food.

To treat diabetes, the research clearly demonstrates that a low-carbohydrate, moderate protein, high-fat diet is effective. For mental health disorders such as major depression, bipolar disorder, and schizophrenia, a high-fat, low-carbohydrate, moderate protein diet is making headway and showing promise. What about a low-carbohydrate, high-fat, moderate protein diet for individuals with eating disorders?

To demonstrate my point, I think it is essential that we look at some of the current statistics with regard to eating disorders. A review of mortality on mental illness found that eating disorders were associated with one of the *highest risks of premature death of any psychiatric disorder.* Without treatment, up to 20% of people with serious eating disorders will die. (18) A sobering statistic is that many individuals with eating disorders do not actually die from medical complications, they die from suicide. One study found that over 11% of individuals with an eating disorder had attempted suicide and 43% experienced suicidal ideation. (19)

Anorexia has one of the highest mortality rates of all psychiatric disorders, including major depression. The mortality rate associated with anorexia is 12 times higher than the death rate of all causes of deaths for females aged 15-24. More females ages 15-24 die from anorexia than illness, car accidents, or any other cause. Indeed, it makes sense that several studies have reported that lower weight, which is a characteristic of anorexia, increases the risk for fatal outcomes. (4,20)

A metanalysis of 36 published studies looking at death rates of patients with anorexia and other eating disorders found that 20% of individuals who died of anorexia took their own lives. (21) Perhaps even more distressing is that 20% of individuals who did survive the physical and mental complications of anorexia remained chronically ill until the end of their lives. Many individuals who suffer from eating disorders find themselves unable to break the chains of their disease. They end up spending their entire existence in and out of hospitals and treatment facilities.

As you read in my personal story, my relationship with food has been the definition of rocky. I attempted to find solace in gluten-free diets, paleo diets, vegan diets, vegetarian diet, and what I like to call, "F*%k it, leave me alone, I'm going to eat anything I want" diets. For the most part, these ways of eating led to more stress and anxiety.

As much as I wanted to believe and embrace that the key to recovering from anorexia would be to "be able to eat anything and everything," to make peace with food, there is evidence that certain foods may prevent our brains from healing and functioning optimally. If certain foods are potentially harmful to our bodies and brains, should they be routinely included in our diets?

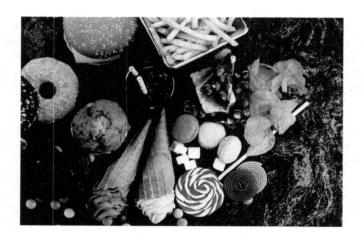

There are foods that can suppress the brain's ability to engage in neuroplasticity. Neuroplasticity is one of my favorite concepts. It basically means that the brain is pliable, moldable and able to change. In the most difficult times in my life, I keep coming back to neuroplasticity. I have held onto the concept that my brain could rewire, and I could change and heal. I believed neuroplasticity could, theoretically, allow me to feel more joy and less anxiety.

Before we talk about food, I want to briefly talk about therapeutic options and why engaging in therapy is non-negotiable in eating disorder recovery. There are several types of therapeutic modalities available, and it is most certainly out of my realm of expertise to advise which one is appropriate for individuals with eating disorders. While writing this book, I spoke with several mental health professionals who specialize in eating disorder treatment. The consensus for treatment modalities is that each therapeutic modality has pros and cons, and therapy must be individually tailored to the individual's specific needs. The current research for treating eating disorders points to utilizing a multimodal approach. This means that a person will often benefit from utilizing several treatment and therapeutic methods depending on their specific needs. This is key because of the complexity, individuality, and unpredictability of eating disorders.

Cognitive Behavioral Therapy and Direct Behavioral Therapy are preferred modalities, but group therapy, family therapy, and even complementary therapies such as art, yoga, or other methods of self-exploration are components of treatment. Certainly, if someone is medically compromised, they may need to be acutely monitored in a hospital setting to ensure compliance and prevent further complications, including mortality. Most experts agree uncovering and processing trauma is a major factor in ensuring recovery.

Have you or a loved one tried many different treatment methods to work through the difficult emotions and coping mechanisms that have manifested during the process of an eating disorder? Perhaps weight restoration or stabilization was achieved, but you your loved one began to fall back into old patterns of thinking or behaving? Does this eventually lead you or them to act on coping mechanisms that are no longer serving you or them? If so, I believe you owe it to yourself to explore if shifting the way you eat might allow your brain to better process all the hard work being done in recovery.

Can you work through your trauma and begin to effectively shift eating habits without a health professional? Can you do this on your own? Truthfully, I have never met anyone who has been able to do it alone. I have worked with several therapists throughout my adolescent and adult life to process trauma, identify negative thought patterns, and develop healthy coping mechanisms. Having a supportive friend, coach, mentor or partner in recovery is an invaluable tool. I am incredibly grateful for the support of my wife, Corene, and the many great friends and coaches I have had over the years.

The evidence shows that if we want to overcome any mental illness, including working through an eating disorder, we must provide our brains with the right nutrients to heal and rewire. Perhaps even more crucial is providing the correct nutrition to keep neurotransmitters, which are the body's chemical messengers, balanced.

The neurotransmitter glutamate and essential amino acid tryptophan are key factors in optimal brain function. Without these two components, our brains are unable to effectively rewire and our recovery may be hindered. If the brain is not able to rewire, engaging in therapy may not be helpful because the brain may be unable to process new information. It is like the saying, "it just goes in one ear and out the other." If you are given new tools and coping mechanisms but the brain cannot process and store that information, you might be unable to act on this new information in a time of stress. In this case, the new information is effectively useless to you.

Recall from our chapter on mental illness that glutamate is a powerful neurotrans-mitter that is released by nerve cells in the brain. Think of the brain as a car. It presses the glutamate gas pedal at exactly the right rate under normal conditions. When the brain is stressed, it's pedal to the metal! The gas pedal is pressed all the way to the floorboard, and the brain is flooded with glutamate. Extremely high levels of glutamate have been found in the blood and brain tissue of individuals with mood and psychotic disorders, as well as in suicide victims. Individuals with depression have higher glutamate levels than healthy controls. (22,23)

Glutamate levels can become elevated due to inflammation. Some causes of this inflammation are brain injury, traumatic stress (like losing a job, a divorce, etc.), mood altering drugs like cocaine and crystal meth, and inflammatory com-ponents which are abundant in the diet. When we eat the Standard American Diet, which is filled with processed carbohydrates such as bagels, cereal, donuts, granola bars, pasta, sugar from sodas, candies, juice drinks, and seed oils such as canola oil, partially hydrogenated oils, and corn oil, the glutamate gas pedal gets pressed down like you are in a road race. The pathways in the brain are not able to perform their functions when they are overwhelmed with glutamate.

This excessive glutamate activity in the brain decreases brain derived neuro-trophic factor (BDNF). This important factor is the key to the brain being able to participate in neuroplasticity. If the brain cannot participate in neuroplasti-city it cannot take in new information and make change.

If the brain of an individual trying to recover from an eating disorder cannot mold, change, and adapt to new thought and behavior patterns in addition to the stress that comes with making change, how can they possibly have mean-ingful recovery and live a full, vibrant life?

It has been my experience that many individuals who have eating disorders des-perately want their lives back. Many are quite hopeful of recovery. But the rate of relapse in eating disorders is high. A cohort study published in 2016 found the rate of relapse to be between 36-41%. (24) Keep in mind, the study counted "relapse" as an individual needing to go back into a treatment facility. The rate of individuals falling back into old patterns is closer to 100%. I absolutely include myself in this statistic. Even if you learn new tools and thought patterns through a particular therapeutic intervention and you provide your body with calories, your brain may not be able to effectively rewire. This may lead you back to previously wired brain pathways during times of stress and difficulty.

For many individuals with an eating disorders, the brain has been wired towards unhealthy, often self-destructive coping habits. While reviewing research about glutamate, I came across an interesting article about glutamate and cocaine addiction. The article discussed that when the brain was flooded with glutamate, parts of the brain stopped communicating with each other. By keeping glutamate from overwhelming the brain, all parts of the brain worked together. If glutamate did overwhelm the brain, the addict was no longer in control of the part of their brain that allowed for change. It became difficult, if not impossible, for the addicted individual to escape falling victim to relapse. *No matter how motivated or how genuine one's desire to recover might be, they simply could not override their brain's chemistry.* The conclusion of the article was that preventing "excessive glutamate" in the brain was a key component of preventing relapse in cocaine addiction. (25)

As you have read in the discussion above, keeping glutamate levels stable, meaning not too much or too little, is essential in keeping the brain functioning properly. (23) Eating in a way that minimizes inflammation in the brain assists in regulating glutamate. It is fascinating that this way of eating might hold promise for preventing relapse in all individuals dealing with addictions. I am personally grateful that the human body and brain have a tremendous capacity to heal when given the right foods.

Diets high in processed foods often lack vitamin B12, B6, and folate, all of which are necessary for serotonin production. Note that vitamin B12 is found *exclusively* in the animal kingdom. Zinc is another mineral that plays a role in neuroplasticity, and it may help the brain rewire and heal. Not getting enough zinc in the diet decreases the growth and development of nervous tissue and depressive symptoms can follow. Lower zinc status was directly linked to depression. (26) Even if zinc is obtained through the diet, it is important to avoid foods that bind with zinc. You could be eating several foods high in zinc, but if you are eating foods that bind to it, your body will not be able to use it.

Many plant foods contain antinutrients such as gluten, lectins, and phytates. These act like magnets to minerals, including zinc, iron, calcium, and magnesium. We will discuss antinutrients briefly in our next chapter and in great detail in our Plants vs Animals chapter. Maintaining adequate zinc stores may be more challenging than initially thought. Studies have shown that zinc levels are decreased by foods that cause stress and inflammation. Some examples of foods known to cause inflammation and therefore could decrease zinc absorption include refined carbohydrates, sugar, and seed oils. (27,28)

How much carbohydrates, fat, protein, vitamins and minerals any food contains is completely irrelevant if your body cannot actually absorb them. For example, 3.5 ounces of raw spinach has 15% of your daily iron requirements. That sounds

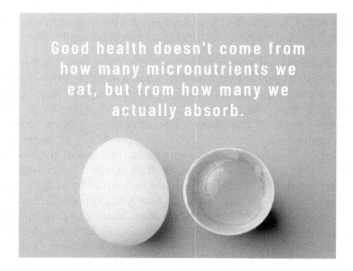

Good health doesn't come from how many micronutrients we eat, but from how many we actually absorb.

great, but the body can only absorb about 1.7% of the 15% of the non-heme iron in spinach. It would be like me writing you a check for a hundred bucks when I only had 17 cents in my bank account. What your body can absorb matters!

For a demonstration on zinc absorption, please note the graph below. If you consume oysters, which are very high in zinc, by themselves, the amount absorbed into the bloodstream is quite high. If you eat oysters with a carbohydrate source such as black beans, the amount of zinc absorbed is significantly less. This is due to the phytates in the beans. They bind to zinc and the body cannot absorb it. Eating oysters with corn tortillas make the zinc completely unabsorbable. This is due to lectins in corn.

Zinc Absorption

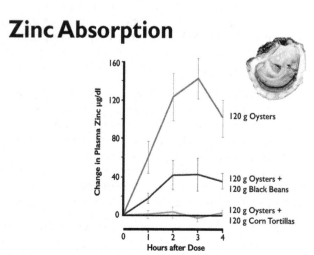

Solomons NW et al. Studies on the bioavailability of zinc in man: II. Absorption of zinc from organic and inorganic sources. *J Lab Clin Med* 1979, 94(2):335-343.
© Georgia Ede MD www.diagnosisdiet.com

I have an eating disorder, so what exactly should I eat?

The number one goal of anyone suffering from an eating disorder should be to ensure that their life is not in danger. If you or someone you love is acutely ill, I encourage you to seek help and explore treatment options as soon as possible. If you are critically ill or suicidal, put this book down and call 911 or your local crisis line.

No way of eating, therapy, or anything else is more crucial than protecting your life.

If you are at a place where your weight is stable, and you are working with a therapist and perhaps being followed by a medical doctor, you could certainly evaluate the pros and cons of following an animal based, high-fat, lower carbohydrate way of eating for a set period of time. Please note this is highly controversial, and you will likely encounter some resistance. Am I suggesting this way of eating will work for everyone that has an eating disorder? No. Am I saying that everyone with an eating disorder must follow this way of eating indefinitely? No. Am I offering an alternative option to fuel your body that aligns with human physiology, can rebuild lost muscle or allow the body to return to its correct weight, and may contribute to the brain rewiring and functioning optimally? Yes.

One of the many reasons this way of eating works well is, in an age where we are under so much stress and life has layers of complexity, it is beautifully simple. The food tastes incredible, it is satisfying, and you will be fulfilling your body's macronutrient and micronutrient needs.

Eating this way can allow you to enjoy great tasting, satisfying food and move on with your life. No obsessing, calorie counting, worrying, planning, or engaging in behaviors. If you had told me six months before I started a high-meat, high-fat, lower carbohydrate way of eating that this was possible, I would not have believed you! Recall from my personal story that my only goal of drastically shifting my eating habits was to help alleviate my muscle pain.

I wasn't looking for peace with food when I found it!

Please note that this way of eating can pave the way for you to heal from an eating disorder or disordered eating. *This is not a substitute for working through the emotional component of why you turned to food in the first place.* That requires a lot of work on your part, and as stated earlier, I believe working with a mental health professional is invaluable. Shifting how you fuel your body sets your body and brain up to be able to process new information, begin the healing process, and move forward.

Several months into eating a diet that closely aligns with human physiology, I was in the bathroom about to pull my hair back before heading out for a run. Like many individuals with an eating disorder, I have made a conscious effort not to look at myself in the mirror unless I am fully clothed. No matter how fit or lean I have become through distance running, I have always viewed my general appearance as subpar. Like many aspects of living with an eating disorder, I came to accept this as something I would need to learn to live with. As I went to put my hair in a ponytail, I caught my reflection in just a sports bra and running shorts. For the first time in decades, I wasn't horrified by what I saw. I felt what I can only describe as an odd feeling of acceptance as I stared at my reflection. Was my brain finally able to make peace with my physical body?

I can't say for sure, but it was a really unique moment that I'll never forget. I can't say I love my body all the time, but I have found peace with food and an acceptance of myself that feels genuine. This is my new reality, and I hope it becomes yours too.

Out of respect, the name of the friend I lost has been changed.

Rosie Lombard

Instagram: @rosie_lombard
YouTube: Rosie Lombard
Podcast: Life with Iain & Rosie (diet, health, and recovery podcast)

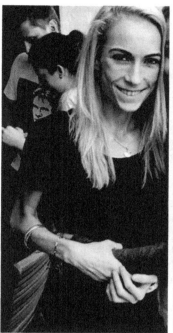
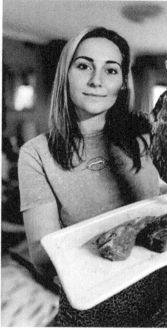

In 2015 I was diagnosed with Anorexia Nervosa. There were many factors that led up to this, but the main issue was never being satisfied or happy with the way I looked. I had struggled for many years, as a teenager, with my weight and really bad body image. I thought that losing weight, exercising more and restricting my diet would help me reach my goals and my 'place of happiness'. To be fair, it did help me reach my goals of being 'skinny,' but I never reached the place of happiness, feeling at peace, or loving myself.

Leading up to my anorexia, I started cutting out different foods such as meat, fats and most carbohydrates. I have always tried to limit processed foods so during my high school career (pre-anorexia stage) I tried to eat as many natural foods as I could, however my body just never responded to anything I was doing. I felt I needed to go to extremes to achieve my goals. Once I left school and was able to make my own decisions, I started heavily manipulating things like diet and exercise. During this stage I was eating only vegetables and very little meat, basically shooting for the lowest calorie foods paired with 3 hours of as much exercise as I could do. This was my routine daily. I started losing loads of weight and with my weight loss came a very bad mental state.

In November 2015 I was diagnosed with Anorexia. The recovery process for an eating disorder is as follows: therapy, dietitians, doctors and eating as much food as possible. What doesn't happen is working on improving food relationships, eating foods that nourish and feed your body as well as tackling the 'sick' mindset that comes along with an eating disorder. Throughout my recovery, I was eating literally the WORST food to try and gain weight. I did gain weight very fast, but I felt so terrible and my body was just in such a bad place. For a few years after becoming weight restored I was in a state of limbo recovery. I was at a decent weight and eating enough but my mind, body and hormones were still a huge mess. I still had a sick mindset and found myself falling into old habits.

I like to say that Carnivore has saved my life, and I truly believe it has! In 2018 I came across the Carnivore Diet and because I had deprived myself from meat and fat, that was literally all my body was craving. Initially, I wanted to try carnivore for the weight loss benefits, still having a terrible mental state, so I did. I haven't lost a single pound of weight BUT I have gained so much more than that! I am over 1 year full carnivore and I finally feel like I am able to let go of my ED, something I never thought I would get rid of! I feel nourished, my body is at a stable weight, my hormones are healing every day and I have regained my cycle. My sleep is phenomenal and most of all my mental health is the best it has ever been in my entire life.

Carnivore has allowed me to restore my food relationships, as I am eating food that makes my body feel amazing, satisfied and nourished. I no longer feel deprived or get huge sugar cravings. I don't feel limited and I am able to eat in public without any anxiety. Carnivore has helped me exile my food rules completely and has made me appreciate what my body has done and is doing for me.

I wish that I had found The Carnivore Diet sooner, but I will forever be thankful for finding it when I did. I am grateful for the amazing community that comes along the diet. I will continue to promote "The Carnivore Diet" especially for people who want and need to recover from an eating disorder. I believe a keto/carnivore diet has so much power and it is amazing just how powerful it can be for someone suffering with a mental issue.

If I could leave you with one piece of advice, it's to give Carnivore a try! Eat as much meat and fat as your body is telling you to eat and listen to what your body is trying to tell you.

Never give up!! I didn't and right now I am rediscovering so much of what my eating disorder took from me thanks to fueling my body with amazing nutrients. I do believe it is that simple!

Jonathan Shane

"Keto helped me find self-love."
Email: theketoroad@gmail.com
Website: https://www.theketoroad.com/
Instagram: @theketoroad

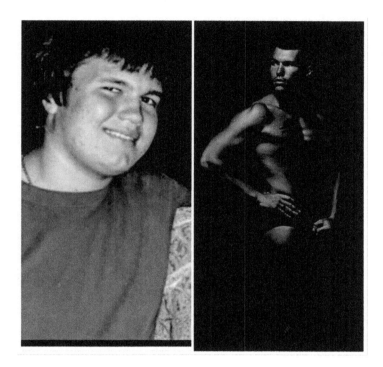

Emotional eating has haunted me since I was a young child. It progressed over time and by the time I was 14, I weighed in at 259lbs. I then began a typical "bro diet" of fat-free ranch, chicken breasts, skim milk and lean protein shakes. I lost a lot of the weight, but I experienced hormonal changes due to lack of nutrition and other physiological/social circumstances. Binges and purges ensued, and I developed bulimia and body dysmorphia. Two years into my journey, I went from 259lbs to 170lbs soaking wet. I was skin and bones, and I throwing up almost every meal. I continued to struggle with this eating disorder and try different diets for the next five years.

In 2017, I came across the ketogenic diet. This diet not only helped me control my eating from a blood sugar balance standpoint, but it helped me in a much deeper way. The foods that tend to come with a proper ketogenic diet (healthy fats, animal proteins and cultured/fermented foods) not only helped with my cravings but they helped heal me from a foundational standpoint. This diet impacted my hormonal and neurological health in ways that allowed me to combat and overcome my bulimia and body dysmorphia. I have now been on a ketogenic diet for three years. I have been in recovery from bulimia and have not experienced a relapse in almost two years. My passion in life is to help those with the same issues as me use a ketogenic diet to overcome them and to help others formulate their ketogenic diet in a way that allows them to avoid those issues all together.

Debbie Wagner

Instagram: @fatfueledat50

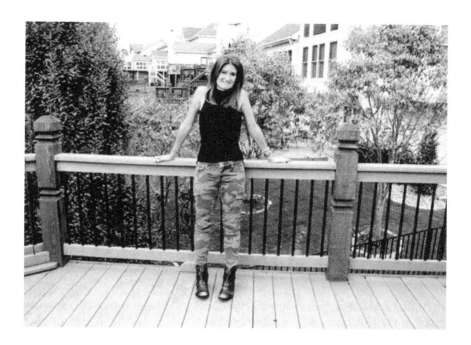

At 50 years old, I was still suffering from bulimia that started in my 20's. At the same time, I began to develop an essential tremor in my hands. I experienced severe pain and bloating every time I ate. Despite trying several diets, I couldn't get my weight struggles under control. While I was never "overweight," bingeing and purging was the mechanism I used to maintain my weight, and I knew that was no way to live. I saw an ad discussing intermittent fasting on Facebook. This led me to the ketogenic diet. I continued to research and learn about low-carb, high-fat diets. After cutting out carbohydrates and nourishing myself with animal protein, I stopped bingeing and purging. My tremor improved, and I no longer experience bloating or abdominal discomfort after meals. I am now following a mostly Carnivore way of eating (high meat, high fat, mostly animal products). At 54 years old I am finally cured of disordered eating. I have never felt better in my life. I only wish I had discovered this lifestyle sooner.

Chapter 4

Sarcopenia: Wasting Away Unnecessarily; A Serious, Preventable Health Concern for Our Elderly Population

There is a belief among many health care professionals and elderly individuals that muscle wasting is simply an inevitable part of aging. "This is just what happens when you get older," is a statement I have heard frequently among elderly patients and many medical doctors in the hospital setting. What causes this progressive, gradual wasting in the first place? Is there *really* no way to stop it or at least slow it down? Throughout this chapter we will explore how our current nutrition guidelines and the recent "plant-based" movement may actually *contribute* to sarcopenia. We will review the current research and statistics on health consequences of muscle loss, the current Recommended Dietary Allowance (RDA) for protein intake, and we will review practical strategies to preserve muscle integrity. We will ask the question: If we follow a diet that aligns with human physiology can we protect ourselves, as well as our parents and grandparents, from slowly losing muscle mass? What if you or someone you know has already experienced significant muscle wasting and weakness? Is it possible to reverse sarcopenia and regain lost muscle mass and strength if we stress our muscles and shift our eating patterns? Let's dive in!

Maintaining muscle mass is incredibly important. Skeletal muscle is an organ that supports the body and enables movement. Recently, it has been discovered that substances produced and released by muscle fibers have an influence on organ systems throughout the body. Maintaining strong, healthy muscle tissue goes beyond the ability to sit, stand, walk, and move freely. Muscle tissue can have a direct, positive influence on organs such as the liver, pancreas, bones, and brain. (1) This means keeping muscles healthy and strong can potentially benefit many areas of the body and keep disease at bay.

On the flip side, skeletal muscle can be broken down due to poor nutrition, underuse or no use at all, and changes in hormonal levels. This breakdown phenomenon is called sarcopenia, a word derived from the Greek words *sarx,* meaning flesh and *penia,* meaning loss. Sarcopenia is defined as a progressive, gradual, subtle disease characterized by 3-8% reduction in lean muscle mass per decade after the age of 30.

Sarcopenia leads to frailty, cachexia (weakness or wasting), osteoporosis, metabolic syndromes, and death. Advanced sarcopenia is associated with an increased likelihood of falls due to weakness. Once a person has advanced sarcopenia, often they are unable to perform one or more routine activities of daily living. (2) Simple, routine activities that healthy individuals are able to do easily and perhaps take for granted become difficult, if not impossible, for these individuals to do without assistance. Some examples of activities of daily living include:

- Personal Hygiene: A person's ability to take care of their own bathing, grooming, oral, hair, and nail care
- Continence Management: A person's physical and mental ability to properly use the bathroom
- Dressing: A person's ability to select and wear the appropriate clothes for different occasions
- Feeding: A person's ability to feed themselves
- Ambulating: A person's ability to change from one position to another and to walk independently

I'd like you to do a quick mental exercise with me. Please close your eyes and picture a person over the age of 65. What image comes to mind? Often, we don't picture a strong, independent man or woman, only identified as aged by gray hair and wrinkles. For many people, the image that comes to mind is much less optimistic. When we talk about "the elderly," often we are referencing a person who has experienced significant physical and mental decline. This person may be obese or underweight. They may not be able to walk or even sit up without assistance. They may have sagging skin, missing teeth, and they might be wearing adult diapers due to a loss of bowel or bladder continence. Having spent quite a bit of time in hospitals as well as in skilled nursing facilities, it is often difficult to tell an individual's chronological age simply by appearance. Most of my elderly patients look significantly older than their true, chronological age due to decades of battling chronic disease.

It is often quite sad to hear stories from the loved ones of these patients. A child or spouse will reminisce about a time when the patient was "independent and strong," but the loss of independence is a heart-breaking reality for many elderly individuals with sarcopenia.

I have often wondered what sequence of events led these chronically ill, muscle-wasted patients to where they are today. How did a person who was once strong, independent, and thriving become so obese and profoundly weak that they can no longer walk, stand, or sit on the toilet without assistance?

The risk of mortality increases significantly once an individual is diagnosed with sarcopenia. This fact alone would seem to signal the necessity to make a lifestyle change once receiving a sarcopenia diagnosis. In a study released in 2013, 67% of patients who were diagnosed with sarcopenia had passed away by the 7-year marker from the diagnosis date. (3)

While I have seen elderly individuals in the hospital setting that are thin and wiry, more often than not, most individuals are obese. We are now seeing a significant, exponential rise in obesity and sarcopenic obesity in our elderly population. (4)

This is no way to live or age, but this is a reality for many Americans as they grow older. Sarcopenia effects 30% of individuals over the age of 60 and a full 50% over the age of 80. (5) The question remains, is this an unavoidable reality? Is this truly an enviable consequence of getting older, or is there a way to remain lean, healthy, and independent until the end of life?

Initially, it might be difficult for an individual or caregiver to notice a loss in strength or muscle mass in an elderly individual. Muscle mass or strength may be slowly decreasing, yet the individual may be gaining fat, thus the individual may not *actually be losing any weight.* (6) The lack of tangible weight loss on a scale may delay interventions that could potentially prevent the patient from suffering the consequences of reduced muscle mass and full-on sarcopenia.

Individuals who have sarcopenia may be underweight, at a normal weight, or clinically obese (sarcopenic obesity.) Obesity by itself increases the risk of the development of high blood pressure, type 2 diabetes mellitus, atherosclerotic heart disease, and stroke. Elderly individuals with sarcopenic obesity have *a higher risk of developing metabolic syndrome* than elderly obese individuals without sarcopenia. (7)

This demonstrates that preventing disease is not just about weight. When an individual begins to lose muscle tissue and bone density while at the same time gaining fat mass, they are at a much greater risk of developing diabetes or heart failure than an individual at the same weight with more muscle and bone and density and less fat. The take-home message is that you want to have strong bones and dense muscles with just enough body fat. What we are seeing in many of our elderly patients, and what I observed daily in the hospital setting, is patients with porous bones, lack of muscle, and excessive body fat.

While more research is needed in this area, these conclusions demonstrate that muscle mass can potentially be protective when it comes to chronic disease. Studies have shown that more muscle mass was consistently associated with reduced mortality. Individuals with more muscle mass demonstrated a greater ability to care for themselves as well as less prevalence of chronic disease. (8)

Patients who are diagnosed with sarcopenia have much higher rates of falls and subsequent broken bones. Elderly patients who fall and suffer a bone break have very poor outcomes. A recent study demonstrated that patients who broke a hip had a 14-58% increased chance of mortality one year after the break. This is due to the effect the break has on the patient's mobility and the difficulty they experience returning to their previous state of health and independence. (9-18)

Losing skeletal muscle as we age has physical, emotional, and financial consequences. In the United States, sarcopenia has been estimated to have an economic burden of $18.5 billion per year related to health care expenditures. Once a person can no longer perform routine activities of daily living, they will likely need a caregiver or they may need to live in a facility where they are completely dependent on others. Among the population age 65+, 69% will develop disabilities before they die, and 35% will eventually enter a nursing home. In 2012, total spending (public, out-of-pocket, and other private spending) for long-term care was just over $219.9 billion, or 9.3% of all U.S. personal health care spending. This is projected to increase to $346 billion by 2040. (19) While nursing home and care giver expenses are not solely related to sarcopenic muscle wasting, sarcopenia and the decline of health from sarcopenia related issues contribute to a large portion of this cost.

What about the emotional toll of lost independence caused by muscle wasting due to sarcopenia? Recall from our chapter on mental illness, that the rate of depression among adults and adolescents is increasing exponentially. In the elderly population, clinical depression is becoming more common. It is estimated that over 6 million individuals over the age of 65 are clinically depressed, but less than 3% will receive treatment from a mental health professional. (20) Depression in the elderly is associated with an increased risk of heart disease and dying from an illness. Depression also reduces the elderly patient's likelihood of fully rehabilitating after a fall, stroke, or major disease. Sarcopenia can set a deadly cycle in motion: over time, an individual loses muscle and gains fat. They suffer a fall and break a hip. Then, the pain and immobility cause them to experience sadness, anger, and feel unimportant. While processing these emotions, they are faced with a loss of independence. This can potentially lead to a loss of purpose. Clinical depression may prevent the elderly individual from fully participating in rehabilitation activities which are designed to help them regain strength and become as independent as possible.

In my years working in the hospital, I have had dozens of elderly individuals tell me they felt lonely, unimportant, anxious, and depressed. Many expressed minimal motivation to heal and rehabilitate, and several of my patients expressed a desire to end their lives.

Current research related to sarcopenia is targeting the mechanisms to help understand how this process begins. Why are individuals over the age of 30 losing muscle mass at such an accelerated rate? As I reviewed the research on sarcopenia, it became clear to me that it is possible to avoid muscle wasting with food and movement. I researched historical accounts of elderly individuals hunting, fishing, and performing manual labor into their late 90's. I viewed stories of body builders and endurance athletes competing at the ages of 82, 96, and as old as 102! If individuals are capable of thriving into advanced age, why are we seeing a massive shift towards disability in the middle-aged population over the last several decades?

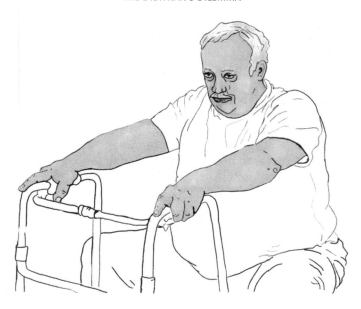

To answer this, we will begin by looking at the dietary trends over the past few decades. We will ask the question, can a diet that aligns with human physiology prevent and even reverse sarcopenia?

As I reviewed the research on sarcopenia, two common themes emerged. The first theme is that sarcopenia is directly tied to the food we eat, specifically protein, and the foods we eat with or instead of protein. The amount and quality of the protein we eat becomes *crucial* as we age. It is quite possible to "get away with" eating less total protein and low-quality protein sources in our teenage years and even into our twenties. Continuing this trend into our thirties and beyond may have disastrous consequences.

The second theme deals with movement. Stressing the muscles activates hormones responsible for ensuring they stay strong and able to perform their functions. Stressing muscles may contribute to the health of other organ systems in the body including the liver, pancreas, and brain. Let's begin by talking about protein.

Protein Intake:

The word protein comes from the Greek word *proteus*, which means "of first importance." Make no mistake, eating high quality, bioavailable protein designed for human consumption is essential to live a full, vibrant life, free of muscle wasting and other chronic ailments. Most individuals understand that protein is necessary for building and maintaining muscle, but that is just one of the many functions of this macronutrient. Protein participates in many biochemical reactions, is responsible for making hormones, provides our cells with structure, and is an essential part of the immune system. As a macronutrient, the many functions of protein continue to amaze me. Science professionals continue to uncover additional functions of protein in the human body.

Since protein has so many essential functions in the body, it is essential to consume adequate protein. If you do not consume adequate protein, your body will break down muscle tissue to keep hormones stable, neurotransmitters firing, your cells intact, and your immune system fighting. Taking in less than adequate amounts of protein can affect many of the body's systems. Muscles become weak, the immune system becomes susceptible to infection and hormone levels can drop rapidly. Recall that the brain requires amino acids to function properly. Individuals with inadequate protein intake are more likely to suffer from anxiety and depression due to lack of precursors to make serotonin and dopamine. (21)

Currently, there is a movement encouraging people to consume a low-quality protein, "plant-based" diet. I feel confident stating that this way of eating will directly contribute to sarcopenia. *Under no circumstances should we encourage individuals to avoid animal protein or eat low bioavailable, poorly digested vegetable proteins.* While a well-meaning, health-motivated individual may think eating more plants and avoiding meat will contribute to health, the opposite is likely to occur.

Focusing on adequate whole food protein intake represents one of the few clinically proven methods to slow or prevent muscle protein breakdown. In the Health, Aging, and Body Composition study, persons who had the highest protein intake lost nearly 40% less muscle mass than persons with the lowest intake. (22) Protein muscle synthesis, which is the naturally occurring process by which protein is utilized to repair and rebuild muscle tissue, is regulated by a host of factors. One of the main factors contributing to protein muscle synthesis is consuming an adequate supply of essential amino acids. This can be done by eating high-protein animal foods. How much protein do you need to eat to maintain a healthy amount of muscle mass? For all men and women aged 18 years and older, the current recommended daily intake (RDI) for protein is 0.6-0.8 grams per kg. This recommendation is the Academy of Nutrition's guideline, and it is designed to prevent disease and death in the *best* of circumstances. For aging individuals with higher nutrition and protein needs, this standard desperately needs to be revisited and increased.

What does the current RDI value look like in real life? For a 150-pound (68 kg) person, getting "adequate" protein to meet the bare minimal standard can be accomplished by simply eating 2 hardboiled eggs in the morning, a 3 oz (about the size of a deck of cards) grilled chicken breast for lunch, and a large portion of vegetable protein like beans or lentils for dinner. These recommendations were originally established by the Institute of Medicine, and they are based on short duration nitrogen balance studies in young adults.

I do not think it makes sense to use the same protein recommendations for the elderly, knowing they experience accelerated muscle breakdown, as we do for healthy, young adults. In my view, and evidenced by the skyrocketing rates of sarcopenia, I believe we should reevaluate the minimal protein requirements for the elderly population.

Just how good are the elderly when it comes to meeting the current RDI recommendations? Are they at least able to obtain this relatively small amount of protein with their daily food choices?

Statistically, they aren't doing very well. Currently, 15-38% of older men and 27-41% of older women fail to meet the current, minimal protein requirements. (23) Recall this is the amount of protein for healthy, young individuals to prevent disease and death. This number does not reflect the increased protein need required to prevent sarcopenia.

Protein intake, and how efficiently the human body can use protein, appears to decrease with age. This means as we get older, not only are we eating less protein, our bodies are not able to effectively use all the protein we do eat. It's a double whammy. Many experts agree that protein intake requirements need to be revisited and updated. Experts have argued that while the RDI for protein may represent the bare minimum amount to prevent disease in healthy, young individuals, it is significantly too low to promote optimal health or protect elders from sarcopenic muscle loss. (22, 24-26) Some studies suggest that a moderately higher protein intake of 1.0-1.3 grams per kg may be required to maintain nitrogen balance and offset a potentially lower energy intake, decreased protein synthetic efficiency, and impaired insulin action in elderly individuals. (22, 25-28)

To recap, while studies are showing that the elderly are failing to even consume the bare minimal protein requirements designed for young healthy people, they actually need to consume *more* than the minimal standards to prevent sarcopenia.

Protein Quality:

Not all protein sources are created equal, and we have evidence that the type of the protein consumed matters when it comes to preventing muscle breakdown. Animal proteins are considered *complete proteins* because they have all the essential amino acids present in the exact ratios that the human body needs to properly absorb and utilize them. This fact alone seems to demonstrate that humans are designed to eat protein from animal sources. Protein from animal sources come packed with highly absorbable vitamins, minerals, and bioactive substances. Animal proteins contain all fat-soluble vitamins (D, E, A, and K), as well as the B vitamins, iron, zinc and phosphorus. There are several key nutrients in the animal kingdom that are difficult, if not impossible, to obtain from plants. Some examples of these nutrients include EPA and

DHA, vitamin B12, vitamin A1, vitamin D3, heme iron, and collagen. Protein sources such as red meat and whey protein are especially high in the amino acid leucine. This could be critical in the efforts to prevent sarcopenia because emerging research indicates that leucine may have a greater stimulatory effect on muscle protein synthesis than any other essential amino acid. (29) Knowing that animal proteins provide all the amino acids, vitamins, and minerals needed to build strong muscle tissue and prevent muscle wasting, it seems to be a disservice to our seniors to steer them away from satisfying beef stews and steaks, and steer them towards processed soy, hemp, or quinoa burgers.

"HEALTHY" DIET

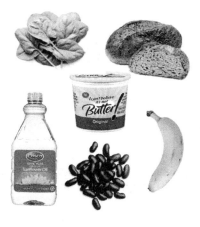

Based on nutrient poor foods

High sugar and high carb

High in antinutrients (lectins)

ANIMAL-BASED DIET

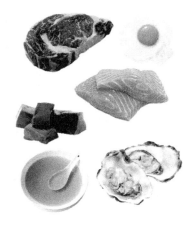

Based on nutrient-dense foods

Low carb means stable energy

Low in antinutrients

Aging is associated with an inability of muscle tissue to respond to low doses of amino acids. (30) This is a crucial and often overlooked point when we are looking at what is the best foods to feed our elderly population. Protein sources from the plant kingdom contain *incomplete proteins*. These proteins are missing essential amino acids. While eating foods with incomplete proteins may have prevented muscle breakdown in adolescence and early adulthood, these same foods become increasingly ineffective at preventing muscle breakdown as we age. The teenager who lived on peanut butter and jelly sandwiches and white flour pasta with tomato sauce may suffer no ill effects from these foods. As this teenager becomes an older adult, they may find their muscles deteriorating rapidly if they continue to eat those same foods low in complete protein.

If this incomplete, low quality protein cannot prevent muscle breakdown, how on Earth could we expect it restore lost muscle tissue? The good news is that high doses of amino acids have been shown to stimulate muscle in the elderly to a similar extent as they do in younger individuals. (31,32) This means while we may not be able to help our elders become stronger and restore lost muscle with peanut butter, tofu, and quinoa patties, we can protect them from muscle loss and even assist in muscle gain with animal proteins such as beef, eggs, cheese, and whey. Animal proteins work perfectly and synergistically in the human body. When it comes to preventing the debilitating condition of sarcopenia, why would we feed our elderly something that is significantly less efficient and, in many cases, less effective?

As stated above, many vegetable proteins are very poor in essential amino acids. The amino acids that are in vegetables tend to have a low bioavailability, meaning they are poorly utilized by the human body. This is a double whammy for individuals that believe they can get all their protein from vegetable sources. Not only are vegetable sources poor in quality protein, the protein they do contain is poorly absorbed and utilized by the human body. Unfortunately, many plant-based, high-protein foods and drinks have clever marketing tactics. These plant-based proteins are often touted as "pure," "clean," "alive," "environmentally friendly," and "the best source of nutrition for the body." Generally, there is no science behind these claims. To maintain and rebuild muscle tissue as we age, our physiology requires high quality animal protein. The best sources are grass fed beef, lamb, bison, venison (or other wild game), pork, dark meat chicken (or other fowl), and organ meats. Whey protein is a great source of amino acids, but I will always advocate for whole foods first.

Many plants contain compounds called antinutrients. Antinutrients further prevent the absorption of the protein in plants, and they can impede the absorption of many minerals in the human body. It is interesting that foods universally accepted as "good for you" can potentially be harmful for some individuals.

Due to the various chemical compounds in plants, many individuals experience autoimmune reactions from eating them, including bloating, itching, stomach pain, headaches, gas, joint pain, inflammation, and much more.

Am I telling you to never eat plants again? Of course not. Though I will note that many people thrive off a plant-free, high-fat, animal-based diet. I am advocating for plants to become a small part of the overall diet *based on individual tolerance*. Humans evolved because we consumed meat and fat. In my view, plants should be eaten on a, "What can I tolerate without harm?" basis. Instead, many people eat plants with an "As many as possible!" mentality. This view has contributed to various autoimmune conditions, like bloating, and the crowding out of nutrient-dense animal foods in our everyday nutrition.

Many vegans, vegan doctors, and health care providers like to tout anti-cancer, anti-inflammatory, antioxidant creating, full body cleansing, "magical" effects of vegetables. Sorry: most of vegetables' beneficial, protective mechanisms do not occur in the human body. Yes, plants have powerful compounds that have been shown to destroy free radicals and theoretically prevent damage and inflammation when tested in petri dishes and test tubes. The human body is not a petri dish or a test tube. As this book teaches, the human body was designed to carefully and effectively utilize the macronutrients and micronutrients present in animal proteins and fats. That is what our genetics and physiology are designed to effectively and efficiently process. Overall, we are very ineffective at utilizing calories, vitamins, and minerals from plant materials.

To wrap up our plant and vegetable discussion, I'd like to ask you a question: Would you sit down and eat a raw head of finely chopped kale, cabbage or broccoli? Would anyone want to sit next to you for hours afterward if you did? Vegetables from the cabbage family contain high amounts of raffinose and fiber, which can lead to abdominal pain, bloating, and severe gas. Do you think your elderly grandmother would rather have a serving of tender, slow-cooked beef with butter, or a pile of steamed broccoli, plain white rice, and a quinoa patty? Would your Grandpa rather have chicken thighs pan fried in tallow, or a raw kale, olive oil, and lentil salad? Most of us eat more starchy plants and vegetables than we probably would if we understood the potential negative health ramifications.

The elderly population tends to be deficient in many nutrients, including B vitamins, iron, zinc, and calcium. These are several of the nutrients that are pulled out of absorption by the antinutrient phytic acid. Phytic acid is defined as a natural substance found in plant seeds that impairs the absorption of zinc, calcium, and iron and has been known to cause mineral deficiencies. (33) Phytic acid is found exclusively in the plant kingdom and exists in foods such as beans, nuts, wheat, rice, oats, and seeds. We can mitigate some of the mineral-robbing effects of phytic acid by soaking, fermenting, or sprouting these foods. How often is the food our elderly population consumes sprouted, soaked, or fermented? Does your elderly grandparent eat store bought whole wheat toast with peanut butter, or do they eat sprouted bread with soaked and sprouted chia seeds? Let's play devil's advocate and say an elderly individual decides to carefully soak and sprout *all* grains, nuts, rice, oats, and seeds they eat. While the soaking and sprouting will prevent *some* of phytic acid's mineral removal, there is another important factor to consider. As individuals age, their overall appetite tends to decrease. With a decrease in appetite, elderly individuals can suffer if nutrient-dense, bioavailable nutrition is not prioritized. (34) If an elderly individual is taking in less volume of food, it makes sense that the food they eat should be as high as possible in absorbable vitamins and minerals as well as contain a complete amino acid profile. This also means that the macronutrient protein must become the first priority in the fight to protect muscle mass. I believe it is a mistake to ask an elderly individual to consume starchy or non-starchy plant foods at the expense of high-quality protein and fat dense animal foods. *The message I'm advocating for our elderly is to eat your beef, pork, salmon, lamb, or chicken thigh first. Then, if your body can tolerate them without any issues, enjoy a small amount of plant foods.*

This information is not widely available or understood in the hospital setting. It is not unusual for a patient in the hospital to start the day with a bowl of high sugar fruit, such as a banana and grapes, oatmeal with brown sugar, toast with jam, and coffee with sugar and creamer. This carbohydrate heavy typical hospital breakfast contains around 10 grams of poorly bioavailable protein, from oatmeal and toast, and between 75-125 grams of carbohydrates! Contrast that with an animal-based, high protein breakfast consisting of 3 pieces of bacon, a cheese omelet, and a cup of coffee with half and half. This breakfast will contain less than 10 grams of carbohydrates and between 25-35 grams of highly absorbable protein, depending on the size of the omelet.

An individual in the hospital might order a tomato soup and a small salad thinking they are being "good" instead of a hearty serving of high-fat beef, pork, or an oily fish like salmon. *Many nutrition and medical professionals have made the mistake of teaching patients that eating low animal protein, low-fat, high carbohydrate-based meals is a good way to resume and maintain health.* They are essentially blaming a modern problem, such as obesity, sarcopenia, or diabetes, on a primitive food (high-fat meat).

How is an elderly individual supposed to meet their protein needs when they fill up on low-fat, highly processed carbohydrates? Often, elderly patients will use high sugar or flour-based items like gravy, or jam, honey, and other sweeteners to make their bland foods taste less like cardboard. Does *anyone* like to eat Cream of Wheat or Cream of Rice plain?

How much stronger and more vibrant would our elderly population be if we served them high quality, satisfying meat with fat? What if we served grilled steak with butter, lamb chops with rosemary and a lemon butter sauce, or salmon with cultured sour cream? How would eating in this way impact healing?

My personal observations while working in several hospitals and doing rotations in nursing homes have demonstrated to me that most plant foods consumed by the elderly are dense in carbohydrates. We know from our previous chapters that high-carbohydrate foods can increase the risk of all kinds of health problems, including diabetes and heart disease. When reviewing ordering trends for elderly patients, a clear trend emerged. The elderly patients were consuming a high percentage of overall calories from wheat, in the form of bread, muffins, donuts, pasta, and desserts, as well as potatoes in the form of hash browns, french fries, potato chips, and mashed potatoes. Although not consumed as frequently as wheat and potatoes, rice, fruit and fruit juices were consumed on a regular basis. These high-carbohydrate, high sugar, nutrient-poor foods tend to crowd out the high-protein, nutrient-dense foods essential for muscle maintenance and overall health.

Would it surprise you to know that an elderly individual on a general diet can order potato chips and a milkshake for breakfast, lunch and dinner in many hospital settings? It is not unusual for an elderly individual to only eat one or two meals per day and then proceed to snack on processed, highly palatable, sugar filled foods, such as cookies, graham crackers and pudding. It seems that it might be a better option to provide one or two high protein, high fat, nutrient-dense meals instead of several small, high carbohydrate meals and snacks. Take a look below at look below at an actual hospital meal vs a high protein, high fat potential meal.

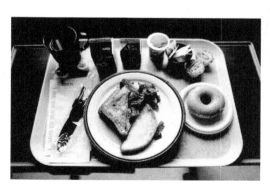 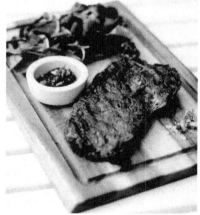

One of the worst things to happen to the aging population is a movement away from animal protein and an increase in protein poor, high-carbohydrate "grain protein" sources such as beans, legumes and rice. Look at the graph provided to see how much less bioavailable animal proteins are compared to plant proteins.

Protein Source	Bio-Availability Index
Whey Protein Isolate Blends	100-159
Whey Concentrate	104
Whole Egg	100
Cow's Milk	91
Egg White	88
Fish	83
Beef	80
Chicken	79
Casein	77
Rice	74
Soy	59
Wheat	54
Beans	49
Peanuts	43

For the majority of older adults, the most practical means for increasing muscle protein synthesis is to simply to have a moderate serving of high biological protein at each meal. It has been suggested that having 25-30 grams of a high biological value protein is a useful strategy to maintain muscle mass and prevent sarcopenia. Recent data has shown that a moderate amount of intact protein, such as a 4 oz serving of beef, contains sufficient amino acids to increase muscle protein synthesis by approximately 50% in both young and elderly men and woman. Currently, experts in the field of nutrition have advocated to increase the RDA for protein for the elderly population from 0.6-0.8 grams per kg to 1.0-1.3 grams per kg.

Would it be beneficial to increase the recommended intake of protein for the elderly even higher than 1.0-1.3 grams per kg? There is little evidence to suggest that protein intake in excess of 2 grams per kg has any negative effects on healthy individuals. One exception might be for individuals with end-stage renal (kidney) failure.

What you eat *with* protein might matter.

What about those very popular boxed protein drinks? Often, these are advertised as nutritionally complete meal replacements. I cringe when I look at the ingredients and sugar content of boxed "meal replacement" drinks. They often have soy protein, followed by sugar, brown rice syrup, and an array of artificial vitamins and minerals. These drinks may have even more sugar than what is listed on the label. Even though it causes your blood sugar to rise higher than table sugar, ingredients like brown rice syrup are not required to be counted as "sugar" on nutrition labels. It's simply a labeling loophole.

Do these drinks provide calories and some protein? Yes, they absolutely do. My concern is, what nutrient-dense foods are crowded out due to the elderly individual drinking 8-12 ounces of sugary soy water every day? In my experience working in the hospital setting, many elderly individuals would consume these highly processed drinks instead of eating real, whole foods. While this may not be a problem for a short time or a specific purpose, it can easily turn into a less than ideal daily habit.

Now that we've reviewed the key component of nutrition, I'd like to segue into the second component to preventing sarcopenia, which is exercise. I'll break the exercise portion down into two separate components, aerobic exercise and anaerobic exercise.

In my experience, just mentioning the word "exercise" can bring about feelings of fear, anxiety, and inadequacy. Many individuals have attempted some bout of strenuous exercise only to become painfully sore, injured, or burnt out. Exercise is meant to provide a *manageable* stress to the system so the system can rebuild and become stronger. The word *manageable* is important because overstressing the system is counterproductive. Exercise should be viewed as enjoyable, challenging, and uplifting.

How much exercise do elderly adults need in order to gain muscle and reduce the risk of sarcopenia? The current recommendation from the CDC advocates that adults 65 years of age and older participate in moderate to vigorous levels of exercise totaling 150 minutes a week. This can easily be broken up into five weekly sessions of 30 minutes at a time. This amount of activity has demonstrated the ability to preserve muscle tissue. As an added bonus, evidence shows 150 minutes a week of moderate exercise can reduce the risk of chronic diseases such as diabetes and heart failure.

How are elderly adults doing when it comes to getting the recommended amount of exercise to preserve muscle tissue and prevent sarcopenia? The statistics show that 60% of American seniors fail to exercise for 150 minutes a week, and a full 21% report no physical activity *at all* beyond what is needed for basic everyday living. Everyday living was defined as getting up to eat, shower, and sleep. (35)

There are two types of exercise, and they each have important roles in keeping muscles healthy and strong.

The first type of exercise is called aerobic exercise (sometimes referred to as cardio.) The word *aerobic* means *with oxygen*, and it refers to the cellular systems utilized when the exercise is performed. This type of exercise is generally performed at a low to moderate intensity and can include activities such as fast walking, jogging, stair climbing, swimming, or cycling. Aerobic exercise helps prevent sarcopenia because it prevents muscle breakdown within the energy centers of the muscle cells.

The second type of exercise is called *anaerobic* exercise (sometimes called resistance or weight training.) The word *anaerobic* means *without oxygen*. These types of exercise are performed for short periods of time with greater force; thus, they utilize a different metabolic system than aerobic exercise. This type of exercise is generally performed at moderate to high intensity for short periods of time. Examples of anerobic exercise include activities such as weight training, isometric training (which can include pushups, wall squats, sit ups) and resistance band training. Resistance exercise strengthens muscle mass, improves muscle function, and increases muscle protein synthesis. (2) It should be noted that resistance training does not have to be done with excessively heavy weights. Even light weights have been shown to increase muscle protein synthesis as long as they are providing enough stress to the muscle. (2)

With all the benefits of exercise, it is important to ask what is preventing our elderly population from participating in exercise? For the elderly community there are several barriers to exercise including a lack of interest, physical pain, shortness of breath, fatigue, and a disbelief that exercise can improve health. It can be frightening and intimidating for an elderly person, who is obese, weak, or has never done any formal exercise, to step into a gym. Attempting to start an exercise program without any assistance might seem like an impossible endeavor. How different would the health of our elderly population be if, as a community, we took the time to help elderly individuals find a simple activity they not only enjoyed but would happily participate in on a regular basis? In 3-6 months, a person's body composition and muscle structure could start to show improvements.

We've covered four very important disease states including diabetes, mental illness, eating disorders and sarcopenia. Now it's time to answer the critical question around heart health: *Will all this meat and fat make my heart explode?* Keep reading!

Mel Honeyman

Instagram: @mel_eats_meat

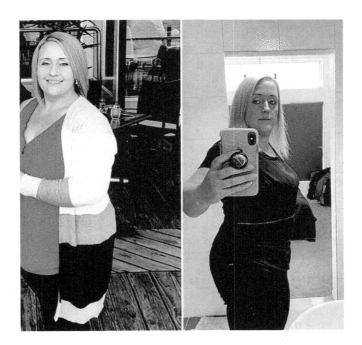

From as early as I can remember, I've been teased by my peers about my weight. I was always heavier than the other kids despite eating healthy and playing sport, etc. My diet as a small child was typical; we used to get fresh whole milk direct from the dairy, ate fresh home-grown vegetables and plenty of meat, but in the early 80's the push for High Carb/Low Fat diet and cutting back on meat meant that mum changed what she was feeding the family.

In High School (age 13-16 in Australia) I played lots of sport (I was House Captain) and I was eating the healthy High Carb/Low Fat diet: lots of fruit and veg, small amounts of protein, etc., but I still couldn't get "thin".

By 18 years old I had gotten to my heaviest teen weight over 100kg. I starved myself and walked hours a day, I cut out meat almost altogether, just some chicken every now and then. I lost weight but I could not sustain what I was doing.

I had my daughter at age 21, and I just ate whatever I wanted during pregnancy. «You are eating for two," people used to say. When I gave birth, I'd put on 25kg, and then I suffered from post-partum depression and gained another 30kg. I never weighed myself so I don't know what my heaviest weight was for that reason. I would try starving myself and then I would binge on carbs. Emotional eating was my way with dealing with feelings and stress.

I found the Atkins Diet after joining the gym to try and help with my weight loss. I had lost a lot of weight already by cutting calories to super low and finally weighed myself at 125kg. Following the Atkins Diet and going to the gym 3-5 days a week, I managed to lose the weight and get to 85kg, the smallest I'd been in my adult life at that time.

Once I went back to a low-fat diet and cut out the meat again, because "Atkins wasn't healthy" according to family and friends, the weight slowing started piling back on. Again, I found myself at 126kg and I couldn't control my emotional binge eating (carbs) and so I did something drastic, I got a Lap Band put in. I was 34 years old. Yes, I lost weight and it was fast, but I was literally starving myself once again. I couldn't keep anything healthy down, or meat, or vegetables unless they were mashed, etc. I was living on iced coffees and chocolate, and most days I didn't have the energy to walk around. I'd fall asleep at my desk. It was terrible! I suffered from severe dehydration and was showing signs of Fatty Liver disease. I was malnourished and deficient in most vitamins and iron, etc. It was killing me slowly; I was at my lowest ever weight of 70kg, but I wasn't healthy, I was SICK.

At 37 years old, my new husband and I decided to have more children. During the first pregnancy, I had to have my Lap Band taken out due to complications, but I managed somehow to only gain 18kg. Our sons are only 21 months apart and the next time the weight piled on. I was about 112kg when I delivered our second son, and I was so upset with myself and my relationship with food. It seemed that due to the Lap Band things had only gotten worse. I was fully addicted to sugar and carbs, and I put on even more weight and was back to 126kg.

I knew I needed to take control over my addiction and that a new Lap Band wasn't the answer. In 2019 I tried numerous times to cut out all the sugar and carbs. I was keto for the whole of that year, but I would continue to fall of the wagon. The sugar and carbs cravings were so strong, and I would be constantly obsessing about food and what I could eat next and what would fit in my macros. It was an agonizing year, and I would lose 10kg and then fall off and gain it all back over and over again. I felt better when I was sticking to keto (my version was low fat, low protein, lots of low-carb veg), I just couldn't control my cravings.

In Nov 2019, I'd had enough of my yo-yoing & my health was concerning. I'd be in pain almost every time I ate, with bloating and chronic constipation. I was getting more and more skin tags, and I had Non-Alcoholic Fatty Liver, chronic joint pain from swelling and inflammation, and headaches. I went to my doctor for advice, and she said my only option was a Gastric Sleeve. She ended up giving me a referral! I went home and cried.

After a couple of days, I thought there must be something else I could do long term that is healthy and sustainable and that stops my sugar and carb cravings. I started researching, and I stumbled across Dr. Ken Berry, Carnivore Yogi, Dr. Paul Salaidino, Dr. Shawn Baker, and others. I binge-watched all their YouTube videos, Facebook, and Instagram stuff and found out that we have all been fed lies about what is truly healthy for the human body and what big companies were just trying to sell to everybody. We have all been brain-washed!!!

I had already been doing my version of keto (which was not the best) for a year but it wasn't helping with my sugar and carb cravings, which I finally acknowledged was an addiction. I decided I'd try Carnivore for the month of January and joined in the fasting challenge with Dr. Berry on the 5th of January to kick start my journey officially.

By the end of January 2020, I'd completed the month and I hadn't cheated once. I was feeling better, I had less aches and pains, I was not feeling hungry and my cravings had been almost fully squashed. I had also lost nearly 10kg, so I said to my husband, "I'm going to keep doing this while I'm feeling great and the weight is coming off."

I'm six months into Carnivore and I've lost 30kg so far and my body composition has changed dramatically. I've lost inches everywhere, going from size 18 jeans to size 14 (Australian Sizing). I mostly now eat OMAD, not because I'm trying to Intermittent Fasting but because I'm just not hungry. I feel like I'm finally in control! My cravings for sugar and carbs are non-existent, but I know I can't have any carbs ever again. For me, if I do it will open a floodgate that will be hard to close. Just like a recovering alcoholic or recovering drug addict can never use or drink again, I can never have sugar or carbs again.

My health is now improving. I no longer have any skin tags, my joint pain is 99% gone, no more headaches, I've reversed my N.A.F.L.D. and have no more chronic pain, bloating or constipation from eating. I have more energy than ever, and I'm not chronically tired anymore. I still have a lot of healing to do in my gut, repairing leaky gut, and getting my hydration/electrolytes back in balance. But I feel better now than I did in my twenties!

I'm still working on other ways other than eating food to cope with my emotional and stress habits but being carnivore has allowed that to be an easier thing to deal with. I can eat bacon or jerky instead of carbs.

My carnivore way of eating consists of mostly ruminant animals, egg yolks and butter (I cut out all other dairy as I was having issues still with inflammation and headaches). I will occasionally have pork or chicken, and if I need to snack, I have pork rinds, beef jerky or biltong. I also drink black coffee, but I'm going to give that up soon to help with my gut healing. I also take vitamin D3/K2 and electrolytes.

I'm finally, after years and years for starving my body and abusing it with sugar and carbs, starting to heal from the inside out. For me, this is going to be a long journey back to complete health and I hope my story helps someone younger who will have the opportunity to heal their body and enjoy a long, healthy, vibrant life before they do lots of damage, like I have done.

I'm looking forward to the rest of my forties being fabulous, and continuing on into my 50's, 60's 70's and 80's being healthy, fit, strong and independent.

Ede Fox

Instagram: @blackcarnivore
YouTube: The Black Carnivore

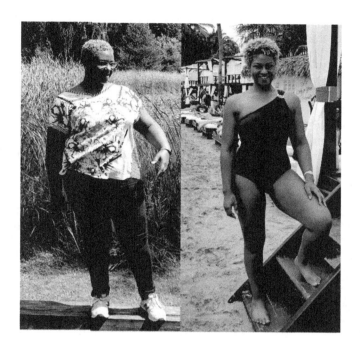

I struggled with weight most of my life, moving from diet to diet, but was perpetually 15-20lbs overweight. I tried low-carb in the past, but considering how addictive sugar is for me, I never made it very long without caving into cravings. I knew low-carb worked for me to lose weight, but it was hard to admit that I couldn't moderate sugar. That ultimately kept me counting carbs and battling cravings just to get a taste of sweets, yet stay in ketosis. I did that for years, then fell off the wagon hard for several years. During that time, I reached a high weight of 246lbs at 44 years old.

At that weight I was swollen, inflamed, and constantly in pain. I assumed this is what middle age felt like and was resigned to my fate. But some part of me got fed up with it and decided enough was enough. I knew low-carb worked for me in the past, so decided to try it again. This time, curious about the science, I immersed myself in all the information I could find. I was fascinated by the information and disgusted that I needlessly battled my biology when I could have been working with it. I believe this is the easiest way of eating, and I am healthier than I have ever been.

By my family's history, I should have high blood pressure, heart disease and be a 300lb diabetic by now. I had terrible allergies, asthma and eczema, my knees and ankles were constantly in pain as well as my feet with plantar fasciitis. Cutting carbs was hard but once I got through it and became fat adapted, I was amazed at how great I felt. Suddenly I had tons of energy, mental clarity and felt happier than I had in a long time. 80lbs later, I knew I had a healthy way of eating that was sustainable for a lifetime.

I had heard about The Carnivore Diet as I searched for keto information but couldn't quite wrap my mind around no vegetables. When I finally gave it a try in December 2017, I knew from day 2, this is how I would eat forever. I loved the food, felt great and more importantly the health symptoms that I still struggled with on keto cleared up. As I lost weight on keto, my inflammation reduced, and allergies improved, but on Carnivore my asthma went away entirely. I no longer use Flonase, Claritin, Benadryl, Sudafed, or my asthma inhaler. No more sinus infections, yeast infections, or bronchitis. I have a level of health now I never would have imagined possible before.

I knew I had to share this miracle with more people, so I started an Instagram account to document my experience. I named myself @blackcarnivore so if any other black people were curious about the Carnivore Diet, they'd find me. I have been inspired by how many other black people are determined to reverse their metabolic disease and achieve optimal health. The community I'm building is growing by leaps and bounds; I've been stunned by just how many black people are thriving on keto and carnivore. I'm so excited to see this movement grow and know that we have the opportunity to live a long and healthy life without suffering the ravages of metabolic disease. I love that discovering this way of eating has helped me build a new and more meaningful career coaching black people into the carnivore way of eating.

Chapter 5

Heart Disease: Red Meat Helps Your Heart Beat

Heart disease is the **leading cause of death** for men, women, and people of most racial and ethnic groups in the United States. (1) Every 37 seconds, someone in the United States dies of cardiovascular disease. (1) Including the cost of health care services, medicines, and lost productivity due to death, heart disease costs the United States approximately **$219 billion** each year. (2) With heart disease causing death and financial burden, it would seem that keeping our hearts healthy would be a top priority for our nation. Heart disease is a national health crisis, yet our current nutrition guidelines, which contributed to the current crisis, remain largely unchanged. Discussed in detail in our chapter on diabetes, the flawed work of physiologist Ancel Keys shaped the nutrition recommendations for preventing and combatting heart disease in America. Currently, in many hospitals, including the one where I practice, a patient on a "heart healthy" diet will have their salt and fat intake at meals restricted, but they are permitted to order unlimited amounts of sugar and carbohydrates.

I'm finishing writing this book during the COVID-19 pandemic. Recently, I lost all of my dietitian hours due to the cancelation of elective surgeries. With less patients to see, I was reallocated to the dietary call center where I was tasked as a call center representative. My new job was taking calls directly from patients while they placed meal and snack orders. I felt my heart drop in my chest when patients on a "heart healthy" diet would order bagels and toast with jam, double portions of rice or spaghetti, juices, high sugar, nonfat espresso drinks, and low-fat desserts. One memorable patient ordered a meal with 87 grams of sugar (over 22 teaspoons).

I reviewed our call center guidelines and attempted to discuss my concerns with my fellow dietitians. Several dietitians were reallocated to the call center, and most seemed happy to just take orders, input data, and move on. As long as patients did not exceed 25 grams of fat or 800 mg of salt per meal, all foods were permitted. During my time in the call center, I heard many representatives argue zealously with patients. They refused to allow them to exceed 800 mg of sodium per meal, and instead they would steer them towards low sodium, low-fat, high-carbohydrate items. It is not uncommon for patients to call in and order up to 150 grams of carbohydrates per meal. *This line of thinking is completely backwards, and it is pivotal in keeping people sick.* Most patients order food at least three times a day, and many order foods up to 6-7 times a day. You might wonder if patients are ordering food for visitors or family members, but recall this is during the COVID pandemic, so no visitors or family members are allowed. Not allowing a patient to order beef and butter, and allowing unlimited juice, low-fat chocolate milk, bagels, and low-fat desserts, made me want to tear my hair out.

Throughout this chapter, we will discuss if demonizing salt and fat has led to improved cardiovascular health. We will ask if restricting salt, saturated fat, and overall fat intake is really "heart healthy" or if these recommendations need to be updated. We will review the role of cholesterol (specifically LDL cholesterol) in the body, and why you may want more of it, not less of it, for optimal health. Finally, we discuss if eating in a way that may prevent heart disease might help you survive the corona virus.

As a young dietitian, I was taught that you could tell if a fat was "bad for you" if it was solid at room temperature. Since saturated fats, such as butter or tallow, are solid at room temperature, they are considered bad. It was drilled into my head that saturated fats would clog your arteries and inevitably lead to obesity, heart disease, and strokes. The best diet to prevent heart disease was a diet very high in complex carbohydrates and fiber. We were taught to encourage *all patients* to eat a diet high in fruits, vegetables, and whole grains, such as oatmeal, brown rice, and whole wheat flour. In 2010, the USDA did a marketing campaign encouraging Americans to, "Make half your grains whole." Food manufacturers jumped on this immediately. Weeks after the campaign began, cookies, crackers, cereals, and even cake mixes boldly advertised how much "healthy whole grain" flour was in their processed product. Inexpensive, blood sugar spiking white flour was replaced with inexpensive, blood sugar spiking whole wheat flour. I remember seeing a cake mix with a big label on the front saying, "Made with 50% whole wheat flour for the health of your family."

On the surface, this line of thinking seems to make sense. Animal fats look very similar to plaque that can clog human arteries. Fruits and vegetables are loaded with fiber which we are told, "binds and carries out artery clogging plaque." It is true that studies have shown that dietary fiber intake can lower blood levels of LDL cholesterol. (3) I worked with a dietitian who informed me it was his "life mission" to make sure every patient he talked to understood how important it was to eat as much fiber as possible.

Throughout my career, I've worked with many dietitians, patients, and medical doctors. Most of these individuals believe that the best diet for heart health has a small to moderate amount of low-fat protein, such as chicken, fish, beans, or tofu, and is extremely high in fiber obtained through fruits, vegetables, and whole grains. This diet should contain as little fat as possible. Often, the handouts we give to patients tell them to use fat "sparingly."

Let's talk cholesterol and more specifically LDL (low density lipoprotein) as it has been deemed the black sheep of the blood lipids. Cholesterol has received a terrible reputation over the years, but it is actually so important that our liver and intestines make up 80% of the cholesterol found in the body *regardless of how much cholesterol containing foods you eat.* Cholesterol is so important to human health that the body makes around 1,200 mg of cholesterol every single day. Cholesterol plays an essential role in maintaining the structure of cell membranes, and it serve as a precursor for making several hormones including estrogen, testosterone, cortisol, progesterone, and aldosterone. (4) Bile acids, which are used to break down the fat we eat, come from cholesterol. Without bile acid, we would not be able to properly break down important fat-soluble vitamins such as vitamin A, E, D, and K. This would quickly lead to us becoming malnourished. Interestingly, when our skin is exposed to sunlight, cholesterol is involved in the process of making vitamin D and a compound called cholesterol sulfate. Cholesterol sulfate has been suggested to play a role in *preventing* the hardening of the arteries. (5)

A great deal of evidence suggests that lipoproteins (such as LDL) may prevent bacterial, viral, and parasitic infections and are an important component for our immune system. LDL may be involved in the process of keeping us from getting sick. Wait, haven't we been told to eat as much fiber as possible to *reduce* this "bad" LDL cholesterol? Haven't we been steered away from red meat, egg yolks, and butter because these foods could possibly raise our LDL and total cholesterol?

A series of experiments were conducted to determine if mice with higher levels of LDL were protected against lethal endotoxemia and severe Gram-negative infections. The researchers wanted to see if they injected mice with a severe bacterial infection, would the LDL come to the rescue and prevent the mice from dying? *The studies showed that mice with a higher LDL were significantly less susceptible to infection and had fewer overall deaths.* (6,7,8) LDL was acting like a bodyguard, binding to various foreign bacteria, viruses, and pathogens and preventing the mice from getting sick.

It would be a missed opportunity not to briefly talk about LDL's role in the COVID-19 pandemic. I work in a hospital where people have come into our ICU, tested positive for COVID-19, been put on ventilators, and died. As a nation, it would behoove us to improve our health to a degree that our bodies could fight the virus. As we will continue to discover throughout the chapter, LDL is the firefighter, the search and rescue worker, the superhero showing up to *save the body from damage.*

A study conducted on patients admitted to the ICU with the COVID-19 virus demonstrated how crucial LDL can be in helping clear the body from foreign invaders, which in this case was the COVID virus. In the cases where patients were able to fight the virus and recover, their low-density lipoprotein (LDL) levels decreased significantly on admission. Their LDL levels continued to decrease during the illness. After the disease was cleared from the body, LDL resumed the original levels as patients recovered. (8) Why did LDL decrease in patients who were able to survive the virus, and why is this significant?

Just like a security guard tackling someone trying to cause harm, LDL appear to be able to do the same with bacteria, **viruses**, and even with some parasites. It's hypothesized that LDL was binding to the pathogen, which in this case is COVID-19, and it blocked the virus from getting into the patient's cells. (9)

Where I live, the news has focused on the number of people dying and the need for a vaccine. While that information is important, I find the minimal coverage on why the virus is infecting people so quickly in the first place unsettling. Are we not less likely to contract the virus if we are in the 12% of Americans who have no metabolic dysfunction and have strong immune systems?

I cannot think of time in recent history where it would be considered crucial to have a strong, optimally functioning immune system. We need LDL and *all mechanisms of our immune system* to be able to perform their protective functions. Obesity, which causes inflammation, and diabetes are considered conditions for, "increased risk of severe illness from COVID-19." (10,11) If you have high blood sugar or inflammation, your immune system may not be functioning as well as it needs to be to effectively fight off infections.

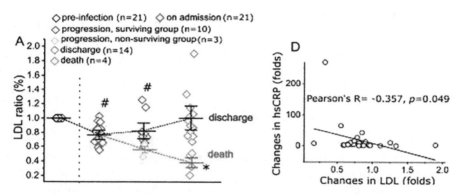

Fan J, Wang H, Ye G, et al. Letter to the Editor: Low-density lipoprotein is a potential predictor of poor prognosis in patients with coronavirus disease 2019. *Metabolism*. 2020;107:154243. doi:10.1016/j.metabol.2020.154243

I'd like to ask you a question. What do you think when you hear the words, "high cholesterol," or "high LDL?" Most people associate these terms with very bad, dangerous things for the human body! Millions of dollars a year are spent on cholesterol lowering medications. Foods such as beans, oats, and some high fiber cereals are labeled touting that they can lower cholesterol. I worked with a dietitian who told me he could never recommend a ketogenic diet because it could raise total cholesterol.

Since LDL has important functions in the body including supporting our immune system, playing a role in breaking down and utilizing fat soluble vitamins, building cell membranes, and assisting in hormone production, *wouldn't more LDL actually be a good thing? On that note, wouldn't eating fiber to reduce LDL potentially be a bad thing?*

There are several studies that suggest higher levels of LDL actually *protect us against infection.* As we age, preventing infection is one component to ensuring longevity. Getting pneumonia as a relatively healthy 20-year-old may cause you an unpleasant week of resting at home and recovering. Getting pneumonia as a diabetic, obese 68-year-old may cause you a trip to the hospital, and it could end your life.

Let's take a look at what the data says. A study involving 347 individuals, all older than 65 years of age, found that low total cholesterol was a significant predictor of death due to nonvascular causes. Those with high cholesterol had half the risk of dying within the referenced population. (12) Higher cholesterol levels were directly related to *elderly people living longer.* This is the opposite of what we are taught in our health care system. This study suggests that simply lowering cholesterol is not the answer to ensuring longevity.

In a large study conducted in the Netherlands, 724 elderly individuals had their cholesterol levels tested over a 10-year period. The results may surprise you. For every 38 milligrams per deciliter *increase* in the participants' total cholesterol, their risk of dying *decreased* by 15%. In their report the authors stated, "In people older than 85 years, high total cholesterol concentrations are associated with longevity owing to lower mortality (less death) from cancer and infections." (13) The author of the study goes on to state, "This casts doubt on the necessity for cholesterol-lowering therapy in the elderly." (13) This brings up a good question about cholesterol lowering medications. Is it a good idea to put all elderly patients with elevated cholesterol levels on cholesterol lowering medications such as statins? Is this necessary?

In studies of patients with active HIV infections, we see evidence that the higher the total cholesterol the lower the risk of mortality. High total cholesterol was directly related to living longer in people with HIV infections. Recall that LDL is proposed to be a part of our immune system that can actively fight pathogens such as bacteria, viruses and parasites. (14)

Let's take a look at two larger studies.

A large meta-analysis looked at 68,406 individuals. The goal of the meta-analysis was to analyze what impact, if any, the total cholesterol of an individual had on the individual dying from an infectious disease. The study found an inverse correlation. The higher an individual's total cholesterol, the less likely they were to die of a respiratory infection or gastrointestinal disease. (15)

In a fifteen-year study of over 120,000 patients, those with the highest total cholesterol had the lowest risk of being admitted to the hospital for an infectious illness. (16)

Finally, in a very large meta-analysis systemic review, which included both observational and randomized controlled trials involving over 600,000 participants, the authors concluded, "Current evidence does not clearly support cardiovascular guidelines that encourage high consumption of polyunsaturated fatty acids and low consumption of total saturated fats."(17) In laymen's terms, getting fats from olive oil, walnuts, or canola oil, instead of butter, tallow, and egg yolks, is not doing your heart any favors.

"HEART HEALTHY" FOODS
THAT AREN'T ACTUALLY GOOD FOR YOUR HEART

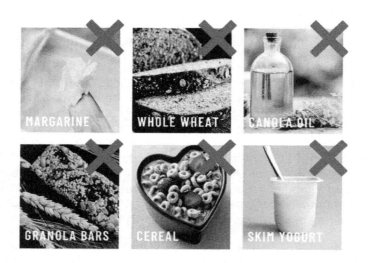

If LDL is a critical component to the immune system, and it appears to actually protect us from infections, why do we find it in clogged arteries? Does LDL have a split personality? Does it protect us from infection one moment then cause plaque formation and a heart attack the next? Stay with me; this is an instance where context is everything.

Most of us drive a car or have driven a car at some point in our lives. Let's say you have a short, 5-mile drive to get to and from your job. Every day you get in your car, drive down the smooth paved road, and park in front of your office. You repeat this process five days a week without any issues.

The car simply delivers you to and from work.

One morning while you're driving to work, you notice your car isn't moving. You hit the gas, the engine revs, but you're stuck. When you take a minute to glance at your rear-view mirror, there are several cars behind you that appear to be stuck as well. After you look around to make sure it's safe, you get out of the car to see if you can figure out what's going on.

There's a super sticky, tar-like substance covering the road. You're going to need help to get your car unstuck, off the road, and back to where it can perform its function of taking you to work. You look down the street and you notice that now there is a very long row of cars completely glued to the road by the tar-like substance. The cars are clogging the road, and nothing can get through.

The car is LDL. It is going about its business, being an effective lipoprotein. It is ensuring we have adequate bile acids, hormones, and protecting our immune system by binding to bacteria and viruses so they can't invade our cells.

Unfortunately, just like our car, LDL can get stuck in arteries and contribute to plaque formation.

This occurs when both LDL (the car) and the arteries (the road) get coated with a sticky substance, or plaque (the tar). When roadside assistance shows up, you wouldn't accuse your car (the LDL) of being the problem! You'd say, *I was driving along and all of the sudden there was tar in the road. Now, my car is stuck to the road because of the tar.* **The tar is the problem, not the car.**

This is similar to what happens in your arteries. LDL, on its own, is not enough to start the process of hardening the arteries. It has to get stuck in the wall of the arteries to participate in forming plaque. In the absence of plaque formation, our heart continues to beat strongly without any issues.

The question we must ask is, *What is causing our arteries and LDL to be sticky, so they contribute to plaque formation?*

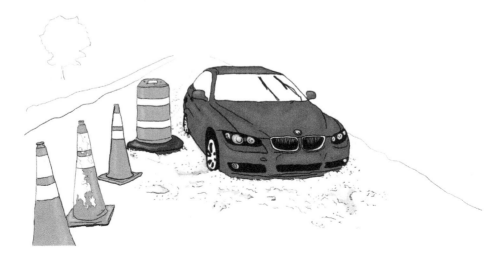

There is good evidence that insulin resistance, which can be caused from eating too many carbohydrates over time, and inflammation cause the arteries and LDL to become sticky. (18, 19, 20, 21, 22) This is one of the reasons that diabetics have an incredibly high risk of having a heart attack. In fact, having diabetes increases the risk of heart disease between two and four-fold. (23) Further, recall from our chapter on mental illness, that the number one cause of death for individuals diagnosed with a severe mental illness is heart disease. Individuals with mental illnesses that are prescribed an antipsychotic medication are at an increased risk for elevated blood sugar and diabetes due to side effects of the medication. It's all connected.

Do you have to have diabetes or insulin resistance to get heart disease? Is it possible to have severe heart problems in the absence of diabetes? Yes, it is. Certain autoimmune conditions such as lupus, rheumatoid arthritis, and ankylosing spondylitis can cause widespread inflammation and damage artery walls. As you can imagine, a diagnosis of heart disease due to one of these conditions, occurs less frequently than a diagnosis due to diabetes and insulin resistance. Recall that an estimated 88% of Americans have some degree of metabolic dysfunction. Many people with mild insulin resistance may not even know it, as they may not be showing any symptoms.

In his book, *The Carnivore Code*, Paul Saladino makes a great point about the relationship between high LDL and heart disease, "If the vast majority of people around us have insulin resistance, is it any wonder that some studies have shown a correlation between (high) LDL levels and cardiovascular disease?" (24) It is not the high LDL levels that are the issue. It is that so many people nowadays have high blood sugar or full-blown diabetes, due to eating excessive amounts of carbohydrates, that their baseline has become the norm. We are targeting LDL when we should be targeting insulin resistance.

It is a huge mistake to look at total cholesterol, HDL, and LDL in a vacuum. This one-sided approach has led to millions of physicians and dietitians encouraging a low fat, low salt, high fiber diet. This has also led to physicians prescribing statins to lower LDL cholesterol.

Looking at this graph below, you could easily make the connection that high LDL increases your risk for cardiovascular disease.

This graph only shows one side of the equation. If you break it down and looked only at the 12% of individuals that are metabolically healthy and insulin sensitive, which means individuals without any type of diabetes or metabolic dysfunction, you would see that *rising LDL does not correlate with increased rates of heart disease.* You must look at things in context.

An article which was released in 2016 showed evidence that in the 1960's three Harvard scientist were paid to downplay the link between sugar and heart disease. There was overwhelming evidence that sugar was the main

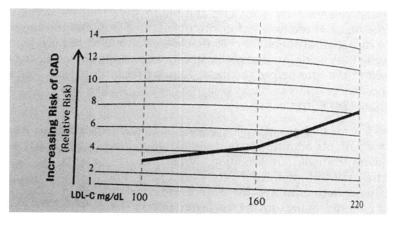

Pic Credit: Gordon, T. el al., (1977) High density lipoprotein as a protective factor against coronary heart disease. The Framingham Study. The American Journal of Medicine, 62(5): 707-714.

driver of insulin resistance and heart disease, so their job was to throw saturated fat under the bus and gently gloss over sugar's role.

The studies used in the review were handpicked by the sugar group. The article cast saturated fat as the main driver of heart disease and minimized the role of sugar. The article was published in the New England Journal, and along with Ancel Keys' flawed research, the invention of high fructose corn syrup, and the many political moves at the time, our nutrition guidelines were designed to be low in fat and high very high in carbohydrates. (25)

Should we be eating unsaturated fat, or can I bring on the butter? A recent study published in the American Journal of Clinical Nutrition wanted to look at the metabolic effects of butter versus olive oil when consumed with carbohydrates.

In the study, participants were fed an 800-calorie meal with 160 calories coming from carbohydrates and the other 640 calories coming from either olive oil or butter. The study wanted to see what effects, if any, consuming carbohydrates with either butter or olive oil might have on glucose, insulin, triglyceride, and free fatty acid levels in the blood.

The study showed that while glucose, insulin, and triglycerides peaked and fell at the same rate in both the butter and olive oil meals, at the three-hour mark, free fatty acids had returned to baseline only in the group that ate the meal with 640 calories from butter. The group that ate the meal with 640 calories from olive oil, had free fatty acid levels *significantly below baseline*.

What does this mean? Three hours after the meal, the group that ate the butter with the carbohydrates had fat cells that were continuing to burn fat for fuel and release fatty acids into the blood stream at the *same rate as before the meal.* Three hours after the meal, the group that ate the olive oil with the carbohydrates had fat cells that were continuing to burn fat for fuel and release fatty acids into the blood stream at a *significantly reduced rate as compared to the rate before the meal.* Burning fat for fuel helps keep blood sugar and energy levels stable as well as allows for fat loss and longer periods of satiation. (34) Butter wins!

I noticed a disturbing trend while working at an acute care facility. As a dietitian, I saw patients admitted to our rehabilitation floor due to burns, strokes, or weakness from various conditions. When we see patients, we look carefully at the types of medications they are taking. I noticed that many of my patients who were admitted for strokes were taking a statin. When I spoke with the patients, many told me they were put on statins to reduce their total cholesterol. Several of these patients had a history of heart disease, diabetes, or both conditions. Over a 3-month period, I kept track of patients admitted for a stroke that were on a statin to reduce total cholesterol. To prevent a HIPAA privacy violation, I did not keep a record of their names or any identifying factors, only birth dates. At the end of three months, I had tracked 78 patients whose ages ranged from 38-77. Over 68% of patients in the group who experienced a stroke were taking a statin. I showed this information to several doctors on the rehabilitation floor. I was told to stay in my lane. The exact words from one MD were, "Come talk to me when you have your medical license."

If you do some research, you will likely see a myriad of articles suggesting that a "low fat, plant-based" diet could reduce heart disease. I want to make it clear that most diets in existence are *much better* than the Standard American Diet. For all the reasons discussed so far and all the reasons we will review in our chapter on plants versus animals, I believe a plant-based diet is a less than ideal diet for your health and the health of the planet. Often when people embark on plant-based diets, they are removing a great deal of processed foods from their diet. If you replace french fries and donuts with an apple and a baked potato, you are likely going to feel better for a short period of time. Removal of meat is not what makes you feel better and certainly these plant foods can fall short in proving absorbable protein and nutrients to your body and brain over the long term.

Talk to me about TMAO

There has been a lot of news about TMAO, or Trimethylamine N-oxide, and its potential connection to heart disease, the key word being "potential." When I was researching TMAO, I found it interesting that articles stated things like, "Those who adhered to paleo had twice the amount of a biomarker that's commonly associated with heart disease than the people who ate a typical diet." (26) This sounds a lot like the frenzy around people eating a high-meat, high-fat diet having "more" LDL than people who eat a low-fat, plant-based diet. You need to take a deep breath, take a step back and ask the question, does elevated TMAO directly cause heart disease? Do we have studies that show that TMAO causes heart disease in the absence of high blood sugar? Let's take a look.

Trimethylamine N-oxide (TMAO) is a small, colorless amine oxide generated from choline, betaine, and carnitine by gut microbial metabolism. (27) As mentioned earlier, choline found in egg yolks and organ meats plays a critical role in the membranes of every cell in our body and is important in neurotransmitter synthesis and brain health. (28) On the same token, carnitine found in red meat plays an important role in energy production, and it gets waste products out of the cells. (29) If choline and carnitine have essential functions in the human body and brain, does it make sense that an amine they create (such as TMAO) would be dangerous for the human body? Some articles have made claims that TMAO causes heart disease in humans, but where's the evidence? Claims that TMAO causes harm to humans is based entirely on observational epidemiology. (30,31) Epidemiology comes down *to observing* diseases in certain populations. *There have been zero clinical trials confirming that HIGH TMAO levels cause any harm in humans.*

When talking about TMAO, many people immediately use it as a reason to eat less meat. "Too much TMAO in the gut! Meat increases TMAO! Eat less meat!" A major problem with this assertion is that TMAO can be produced by the bacteria in our gut when we eat vegetables. (27, 31) Diets of individuals eating vegetables and fish have been shown to be higher in TMAO than those eating meat. (32)

Do you see the quandary here? One of the major problems with epidemiology is that it tries to make correlation equal causation. Epidemiology should be the *foundation to make a hypothesis*. Then, that hypothesis should be tested in a clinical trial. Without doing this, you are simply stating that one thing relates to the other. Check out the graph below:

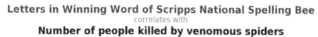

Letters in Winning Word of Scripps National Spelling Bee
correlates with
Number of people killed by venomous spiders

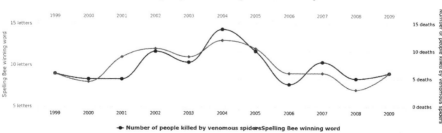

If we took this as fact, we would look at the above graph and determine that the number of winning words directly causes people to be killed by venomous spiders. Most people know this conclusion is preposterous, but that is exactly the kind of conclusions that are drawn through epidemiology. To understand if A is causing B, you ask questions, look deeper, analyze variables, and then you must put your hypothesis to the test.

In a study looking into the role of TMAO in humans, the author concluded, "It is questioned whether TMAO is the mediator or a bystander in the disease process." (27) In other words, they could not tell if TMAO had any negative effects or it was just performing its normal function. Just like LDL, TMAO is doing what it is supposed to do and minding its own business. Zealous plant eaters like to throw TMAO under the bus when there appears to be a correlation between the level of TMAO in the body and heart disease.

If you believe correlation always equals causation, I would encourage you to watch out for venomous spiders if you are attending a spelling bee. This may be especially important if the spelling bee participants have to recite large words. Certainly, there are people who have *elevated blood sugar levels and* elevated TMAO levels who end up getting heart disease, but I'm going to go out on a limb here and say TMAO is not the main problem in this scenario.

Salt: *We got it wrong.*

Just like saturated fat, salt has been demonized. Salt is essential in the human body, yet the government, as well as a myriad of leading health experts, has convinced us that salt leads to high blood pressure, and chronic high blood pressure leads to heart disease. An excellent book on this topic is *The Salt Fix: Why the Experts Got It All Wrong*, by Dr. James DiNicolantonio. Growing up, my family bought "lite" salt because my parents believed salt was bad for you and could cause heart problems. As a dietitian, I have seen patients eat bland, salt-free food, or smother salt-free meals in high sugar condiments or try to pretend that they really do like salt-free herb packets with food.

Is a low salt diet good or necessary? What happens in the body when we chronically restrict salt? Endocrinologists believe that restricting salt causes "internal starvation." The body needs salt, so if you are restricting salt, the body begins to panic. To preserve sodium, the body will increase our insulin levels because insulin allows your kidneys to retain sodium. What happens when insulin levels are high? Not only can you not burn fat, you start to crave carbohydrates like crazy. Isn't that interesting? By restricting sodium, we are setting ourselves up to crave sugar and carbohydrates, while preventing our bodies from burning fat.

Did we have sufficient evidence to recommend reducing salt in the first place? Back in 1977, the surgeon general stated that there was no evidence that lowering salt intake had any effect on blood pressure.

Heart rate actually increases on a low salt diet. Other potential issues caused by a low salt diet include compromised kidney function, adrenal insufficiency, hypothyroidism, higher triglycerides, higher insulin levels and ultimately insulin resistance, as well as type 2 diabetes. Like so many things in health, context is important. If you are eating the Standard American Diet, which is very high in carbohydrates, sugar, and fat, you could see a slightly lower blood pressure by reducing salt. Would this slightly lower blood pressure be worth the negative consequences caused by a low salt diet? Does it lead to a reduction in heart disease? After reviewing the evidence, my answer would be *no*.

I agree with Dr. DiNicolantonio when he says, "It's clear we have been focusing on the wrong white crystal all along."

There is good evidence that keeping insulin levels low combats heart disease. Adopting a high-fat, moderate protein, low-carbohydrate lifestyle can do just that. This way of eating keeps blood sugar levels stable, prevents inflammation, and allows LDL to perform its many important functions including keeping our bodies free from disease. While there are several factors that contribute to heart disease, my experience has shown me that what you choose to eat and choose not to eat is the most important factor when it comes to preventing heart disease. As a nation, we cannot continue to eat in a way in which we have *clinically demonstrated* will cause insulin resistance and expect to reduce rates of heart disease. We will not be able to simply "medicate" or "moderate" our way out of heart disease either.

Recall that for 3.5 million years of evolution, our ancestors ate a diet consisting of mostly meat and fat. Pre-agricultural humans were taller, had minimal evidence of tooth decay and had no evidence of porotic hyperostosis, a condition that affects bones of the cranial vault due to deficiencies in minerals such as iron. (33) It does not make sense that a primitive food, such as high-fat red meat, which was consumed for millions of years, suddenly became the direct cause of a modern disease.

The testimonies in this book as well as my personal testimony show that *dramatically reducing to full-on eliminating carbohydrates and sugars* can have a profound, positive effect on physical and emotional health, and prevent and alleviate symptoms of many chronic diseases, including heart disease. Many of the individuals featured in this book completely transformed their physical, mental, and emotional health with this way of eating.

Did humans eat some carbohydrates throughout evolution? Absolutely. We have evidence that depending on where people lived and what the climate was like, some groups of people ate small bitter fruits, leaves, bark, and tubers. In our modern society, certain people are able to tolerate some carbohydrates quite well while others experience negative physical or emotional consequences from eating even a very small amounts of carbohydrates. In general, processed carbohydrates such as commercial breads, cookies, crackers, pasta, and cereal tend to universally override our ability to regulate how much of them we will eat. In our "Getting Started" chapter, I'll review how to re-introduce plants into your diet. As stated throughout this book, I do not believe everyone needs to follow a zero carb, all meat diet. This way of eating does work quite well for many people and I think it is an excellent place to start. Hang tight, we will discuss this and adding plants into the diet in detail soon.

Phillip Meece

Creator of the Carnivore Bar
Instagram: @thecarnivorebar

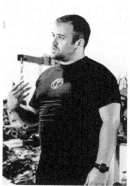 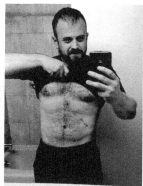 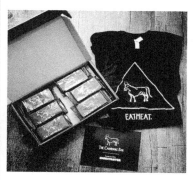

My name is Phillip Meece. I was a combat medic in Afghanistan, a living organ donor, and the creator of a successful Kickstarter. "How are these things related?" you might ask. The answer is simple: The Carnivore Diet. While overseas, I got sick from eating a bunch of sugary preserved crap and also got symptoms of dysbiosis from the antibiotics they gave me as an antimalarial prophylactic. No complaints for Uncle Sam though, I'm malaria free to this day! However, it was quite a long journey to overcome and figure out what was really going on with me.

Early on, about 2012, I realized that what I was eating was making me feel a lot better or a lot worse depending on the quality of the ingredients that I ate. I went Paleo and started investing in grass-fed meat. This helped a little but didn't really solve my issues. I went keto and grass-fed and that helped a little more, but I still struggled with energy and adherence. Finally, I had the opportunity to give a part of my liver to my cousin and dialed in my diet stricter than I had ever thought possible. Truly, the motivation of having someone else's life in your hands is a great dieting tool. I cut all alcohol and all cheats. Just healthy fats, healthy grass-fed meat, and lots of fresh, organic veggies. But I still struggled. Until I heard Mikhaila Peterson's story on Joe Rogan's podcast. So I said, what the heck, I'll give the Carnivore Diet a try. I'm most of the way there already, and voila! Another 20 lbs. came off, I lost tons of inflammation, my mind became clear, and my anxiety vanished. Until that is, I thought about trying to travel with this way of eating. There's no way I wanted to go back to how I was eating, but what can I eat reliably that won't leave me hungry or risk contamination to my newly discovered sensitivities to plants?

I created The Carnivore Bar, which is basically just modern-day pemmican: beef, tallow, and salt. I asked if anyone else would want me to make this for them too, and I had an overwhelming response. We raised $84,000 on Kickstarter and we were off to the races. The rest is history. I hope to continue to provide a safe, reliable pemmican bar for keto and carnivore folks on the go for as long as I am able. I've found my family, my community and my passion all in one.

Rose S.

Instagram: @wild_bk_carnivore_alchemy
Carnivore Coaching: https://meatrx.com/product/rose-s/

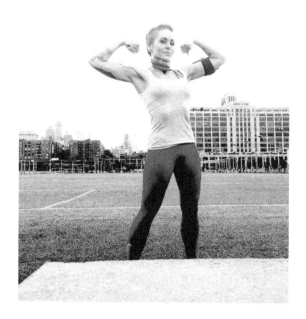

My story really began when I was 5 years old. I remember as clear as day the afternoon my beautiful, amazing mother came to pick me up from school for the first time in months. Her absence hadn't been because of travel or marital issues; she had been bedridden for almost a year due to a debilitating autoimmune illness. It was a joyful surprise seeing her out in the sunshine, standing up, smiling. In that moment, I developed a deep desire to seek out a way to prolong wellness.

I was not a healthy child, and the various red flags that are now commonly accepted as markers of systemic underlying inflammation were all present but not yet identified. I dealt with prediabetes, consistently high triglycerides, anemia, IBS, colitis, interstitial cystitis, fibrocystic breasts, cystic acne, debilitating menstruation, diagnosed depression/PTSD, celiac disease and finally, chronic fatigue/arthritis/fibromyalgia. This last thing resulted in me sobbing most mornings at 24 years old, asking my partner to button my shirt buttons or run my hands under hot water to help them get moving due to the overwhelming pain.

I was devastated and I was angry. I had spent my teen years and early to mid-twenties devoted to a plant-based diet. I had eliminated processed foods and experimented with various elimination protocols, detoxes and cleanses. I was so obsessed, in fact, that I worked part time in the health/holistic nutritional industry for 11 years so I could gain access to training, discounts and cutting-edge supplements. I had guidance from some of the leading lights of the vegan industry, and STILL I was getting worse. I had done everything right! So why was everything going wrong?

Thanks to "the gift of desperation," I decided to try something extreme: I reintroduced meat into my diet. I began experimenting with a plant-leaning keto diet, a paleo keto diet, a modified autoimmune keto diet and, finally, a meat-heavy keto diet. Each step along the way gave me better and better results. This was hard for me to accept. I had been told my womb would rot and fall out of my body or that I would die of cancer from eating meat. So, as the meat-to-plant ratios of my diet began to shift, favoring meat and yielding healing results, I was happy but confused.

In the course of my online explorations, I stumbled upon Dr. Shawn Baker and the investigative research of Nina Teicholz. The Carnivore Diet existed! My heart began to race. Could it be? I realized in that moment that I had been waiting for the other shoe to drop, to be punished for healing through eating meat. But after diving into the mountains of information that revealed themselves once I actually started looking, I realized I was right to intuit that eliminating certain foods and spotlighting others could provide me with the vitality and quality of life I'd always hoped for. I was just focusing on the wrong foods!

I then began a year of strict carnivore and saw almost all of my autoimmune symptoms reverse. Now, 3.5 years in, I'm in awe of the progress I've made and so thankful that my biggest concern now is learning how to manage my emotional state of being. Because as for my physical state...well, let's just say the healing power of meat can make a five-year-old's wish come true.

Chapter 6

Where the *F* Did These Guidelines Come From?

What response would you get if you went up to a random person and asked the following question: *Excuse me, where do you think the USDA food pyramid (now myplate) nutrition guidelines came from?* I would imagine most people might say something along the lines of, "science," or "research" or "health studies." This could not be further from the truth. How the nutrition guidelines came into existence sounds like a bizarre, fictional story with sprinklings of political influence and a few sporadic facts to make it seem believable. As you will see, the creation of the nutrition guidelines has very little to do with health and appears to have everything to do with political power and corporate profit. I find it disheartening that in 2015 experts in the health industry publicly admitted they were wrong about the role of fat and saturated fat in human health, yet the guidelines, which demonize meat and saturated fat, remain unchanged.

Thankfully, we are now seeing a wave of highly educated medical professionals, a few renegade dietitians, and otherwise empowered individuals advocating for the nutrition guidelines to be revised. Unfortunately, many health professionals and dietitians have fallen prey to powerful corporate lobbying. They are on team PepsiCo and team General Mills. Both of these corporations and many others, which we discuss later, funnel thousands of dollars to the Academy of Nutrition, the governing board of all dietitians.

In order to piece together how our nation became one where over 70% of the population is overweight and a whopping 40% is obese, it is helpful to look back into history to see how human evolution began. (37)

For over 3.5 million years humans ate predominantly meat and fat. While experts argue about when exactly humans started cooking meat, they all agree that the development of the human skeletal structure, our increasing brain size, and our ability to walk upright came from eating nutrient-dense animal products.

Plants that were available in primitive history were small, bitter, and very poor in nutrition. Animal flesh, organs, bone marrow, and fat surrounding the organs were dense in calories, fatty acids, protein, and an array of highly absorbable vitamins and minerals.

Humans did eat plants at certain times throughout our evolution, especially when animals were scarce. The fruits and vegetables we consume today have very little resemblance to what our ancestors would have encountered millions of years ago. For example, primitive peaches were the size of a current day cherry, and they were sour, slightly salty, and contained minimal carbohydrates. Carrots were small, bitter, and had white or purplish hues. Primitive carrots had significantly less stored carbohydrates and almost no sugars compared to the large, orange varieties we enjoy today. Bananas grown thousands of years ago contained hard seeds and very little sugar, while today's bananas contain no hard seeds and high amounts of easily absorbable sugar. Over thousands of years, these plants have been cultivated and hybridized to contain significantly more carbohydrates and sugar than they did throughout the course of evolution.

When animal foods were present, there was little need to eat plants because the nutritional benefit and feeling of fullness they created was minimal, especially compared to the calorie dense, highly nutritious animal meat, fat, and organs. There is evidence than humans living closer to the equator ate more plants than humans living further away from the equator due to increased availability.

Humans who lived in extremely cold or harsh climates could go for *years at a time* with minimal or no plant material consumed. While you'll hear a large portion of health professionals and well-meaning grandparents tell you to, "Eat your vegetables," humans not only survived, but thrived, with minimal and sometimes no vegetation intake whatsoever.

If you lived 3.5 million years ago, you had a much higher probability of dying from birth to age 15 than you would today. There was less access to clean water, weaker sanitary habits, and you had to deal with issues like illnesses from poor drinking water, infection from wounds, an unsuccessful hunt, or bad fall. Today, we have excellent access to clean water, and we can treat infections and major illnesses with a spectrum of highly effective antibiotics, antiparasitics, and antivirals. While we excel at treating acute illnesses, our nation is being crippled by a wave of serious, yet highly preventable chronic illnesses. Diabetes, mental illnesses including depression and anxiety, eating disorders, sarcopenia, and heart disease are just a few of the chronic illnesses that plague our society today.

For the first time in the history of humanity, *we are massively overfed yet profoundly undernourished.* Indeed, most of the hospital patients I see are morbidly obese, yet malnourished. These patients, some of which are as young as in their early thirties, have become so overly fat yet have such profound muscle wasting, that they can no longer sit up or stand without assistance. They require two nurses or certified nursing assistants to help them walk the 3-4 steps to the toilet. How did this happen?

Shouldn't our nutrition guidelines be impacting health in a positive way? Shouldn't they be an important part of the solution for the plummeting health of our nation? You would think so. I believe once you understand how the current nutrition guidelines came into existence, it will make sense as to why they will never be aligned with promoting human health.

How do you feel about religion being a driving force for policy? The Academy of Nutrition Guidelines were highly influenced and continue to be driven *by a young woman's vision from God.*

Ellen White was born November 26, 1827. She claimed to have received over 2,000 visions from God over her lifetime. One of those visions involved major health reform. On June 6, 1863, she claimed to have received a vision where God told her that humans were to refrain from "flesh food" (meat). She characterized this vision as, "a great light from the Lord," adding, "I did not seek this light; I did not study to obtain it; it was given to me by the Lord to give to others." (1) Ellen went on to claim, "In grains, fruits, vegetables, and nuts, are to be found all the food elements that we need. If we will come to the Lord in simplicity of mind, He will teach us how to prepare wholesome food free from the taint of flesh-meat." (2) Using only what she claimed was a "vision from God," Ellen professed that meat was not necessary for human health. She stated it caused cancers, tumors, and pulmonary disease. (3) She went onto to suggest that meat created lustful thoughts in men and women and led to the sinful act of masturbation (*Perish the thought!*). She wrapped up her the conclusions of her vision by commanding, "No meat will be used by His people."

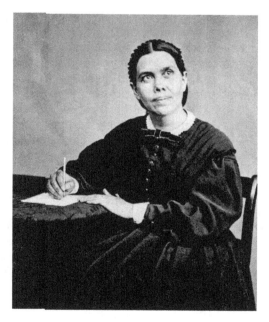

Ellen White Picture Credit: https://en.wikipedia.org/wiki/Ellen_G._White

White would go on to co-find the Loma Linda Sanitarium on April 15, 1906. This building would be used to teach individuals who wanted to be educated in what Ellen White called, "medical evangelicalism." If you wanted to be able to practice "medical evangelicalism" you were required to preach, teach, and adhere to her nutrition and religious beliefs. Ellen, along with other Adventist leaders, such as Joseph Bates and Ellen's husband, James White, was instrumental within a small group of early Adventists who formed what became known as the Seventh-day Adventist Church. (38)

On December 9, 1909, Pastor Burden and other school leaders obtained a charter from the state of California to operate the Loma Linda Sanitarium under the new name of The College of Medical Evangelists. This would be the name by which the institution would be known for more than half a century until 1961, when it became the more current Loma Linda University.

The College of Medical Evangelists was fully authorized to "establish and maintain, carry on and conduct literary, scientific, medical, dental, pharmaceutical, and medical missionary colleges or seminaries of learning." It could grant degrees in liberal arts and sciences, dentistry, and medicine. I find it astonishing that an institution based on "visions from God" and research exclusively conducted under its own roof, was granted the ability to teach medical professionals, including doctors, dentists, and dietitians.

A young man named John worked with Ellen White from the age of twelve and was highly influenced by her visions and teaching. He would go on to become a doctor, inventor, and nutritionist. He wrote extensively on his Seventh-day Adventist beliefs which included following a strict vegetarian diet and practicing sexual abstinence. John concurred with Ellen that masturbation was a "serious sin," and he worked diligently to develop several food items, including the meat analogues, Nuttose and Protose. These meat substitutes, along with a breakfast cereal he created, were designed to be an anaphrodisiac. John's last name was Kellogg, and he was the creator of Kellogg's Corn Flakes. Kellogg's and his breakfast cereal changed the landscape of breakfast in America and helped people start their day with crunchy corn flakes and evaluated blood sugar. (39)

John Kellogg became the director of the Battle Creek Sanitarium, which had been created by the Seventh Day Adventist church and was considered a "world renowned health resort" in Battle Creek, Michigan. Lenna Francis Cooper became the first dietitian of the Battle Creek Sanitarium. She would go on to co-found the American Dietetic Association, which is now known as today as the Academy of Nutrition, and she would ultimately advocate for a vegetarian diet.

It is beyond the scope of this book to dive into John Kellogg's entire life, but it is of note that he spent the last 30 years of his life promoting eugenics and discouraged "racial mixing," while encouraging the sterilization of the mentally ill. (40,41)

Around this time, in 1917, the Academy of Nutrition and Dietetics was founded in Cleveland, Ohio. Upon its formation, the main goal of the academy was to help the government conserve food and improve public health during WWI. Animal products, including meat, eggs, and butter were staples of the American diet, and they were looked upon favorably by the Academy of Nutrition until the late 1970's. I had an elderly college professor who told me, "I remember when whole milk and fatty meat were considered important household staples back in the 40's and 50's."

Back at the Loma Linda campus, a man named E.H Risley was appointed as Dean. It was his responsibility to lay the foundation for the course work for all dietetic students. Risley boldly stated, "Most people have thought that in order to build the body tissues we must have the protein of flesh foods. Scientific men are recognizing the fact that we can get a properly balanced diet without the use of meat. Why should we be so slow in selecting our protein foods from vegetable sources? There is no excuse for the use of meat." (4) He did not elaborate on who these "scientific men" were.

Meanwhile, at the Loma Linda campus two teachers, Dr. Hardinge and U.D. Register, initiated studies on non-flesh diets. They compared the diets of vegetarians with those of nonvegetarians. Their goal was to show that vegetarian diets were superior to diets that contained meat. Originally, the American Dietetic Association was cautious to promote "non-flesh diets." The American Dietic Association expressed concerns that removing meat and animal proteins from the diet could cause vitamin and mineral deficiencies, especially in growing children.

One major concern for removing meat and animal products was vitamin B12. Current science has shown there is no appreciable vitamin B12 in the plant kingdom. There is also no vitamin K2, D3, or preformed vitamin A in the plant kingdom. Most individuals who follow a vegan diet take a B12 supplement to prevent deficiency. This lack of B12 was a big problem for Ellen White and her no-meat followers. Ellen called upon U.D. Register to do "research" to show that her visions from God were true. U.D. Register was apparently quite dismayed when he tested over 100 plant foods at Loma Linda and none contained a trace of vitamin B12. The pressure mounted to confirm Ellen White's vegetarian vision. U.D. Register went on record making the following false, yet plausible to the ill-informed person, statement: "If one eats a very limited amount of refined foods, such as sugar and refined oil, and uses fruits, whole grains, vegetables, and nuts, and eats sufficient to meet his caloric needs, the diet will contain adequate protein. If he does not push his protein intake, no B12 problems should result." (6) *This is not true.*

As staff at Loma Linda University, specifically U.D. Register, churned out and published nutrition "research," the American Dietetic Association began to shift their position on the concept of non-flesh diets. They accepted papers on vegetarian studies beginning in the mid-1960s. In 1988, with the help of Dr. Register and Kathleen Zolber, they published a position paper accepting that vegetarian diets were adequate and wholesome. Towards the end of this chapter, we will discuss the potential conflict of interest within the American Dietetic Association, now called the Academy of Nutrition, who helped publish this paper.

Ellen White and her husband James would go on to write an entire nutrition book with bizarre, unproven ideals called *Christian Temperance and Bible Hygiene*.

I'll go over a few of her statements just to give you an idea of what she was teaching her dietetic students. One example of her ideals is, *"It is a religious duty for every Christian girl and woman to learn at once to make good, sweet, light bread from unbolted wheat flour."* (8) Ellen believed that every girl needed to be able to make bread, and bread should be the cornerstone of every human diet. Recall what item is at the base of the food pyramid, as in, what should be consumed most.

Another example: *"We have on our table no butter, no meat, no cheese, no greasy mixtures of food. Food should be prepared in as simple a manner as possible, free from an undue amount of salt."* (8) White describes items such as meat, cheese, and butter as "greasy" and implies they are "not simple." As you will see throughout this book, meat and fat have the most absorbable nutrition of any food source on the planet, and one of the beautiful parts of consuming meat and fat is their satiation factor and simplicity.

White continues, *"Many a mother sets a table that is a snare to her family. Flesh meats, butter, cheese, rich pastry, spiced foods, and condiments are freely partaken of by both old and young. These things do their work in **deranging the stomach, exciting the nerves, and enfeebling the intellect**. The blood-making organs cannot convert such things into good blood."*

Let's stop right there. The human stomach was designed to be able to efficiently digest meat and absorb nutrients. The human stomach has acidity level of 1.5-3.5. (35) The higher acidity allowed humans to digest scavenged, raw meat throughout evolution. Our stomach acid is similar to that of a wolf which has a stomach acid level of 1.0-2.0. (36) It is *significantly different* than an herbivore, like a sheep, which has a stomach acidity level of 6.4-6.8. (34) The alkaline environment in the stomach of a sheep, goat, or cow allows the herbivore to effectively digest and process grass and plants. Unlike our four-legged herbivore friends, humans need an acidic stomach. This is why taking antacids overtime can cause major health issues. A gut with suppressed stomach acid becomes vulnerable to harmful microorganism such as bacteria, viruses, and parasites. (42) Meat does not "derange" the stomach, it begins to break down protein easily and efficiently.

Finally, White writes, *"When properly prepared, olives, like nuts, supply the place of butter and flesh meats. The oil, as eaten in the olive, is far preferable to animal oil or fat."* Recall that since the 1970's our consumption of vegetable oils has skyrocketed. We are taking in significantly less animal fat compared to our intake in 1970, yet our chronic diseases such as diabetes, heart disease, and mental illness are reaching epidemic levels.

Ellen White did make one prophecy that has come to fruition: **"The health food business... is to supply the people with food which will take the place of flesh meat, and also milk and butter..."** (8) She envisioned the Health Food Industry creating fake meats, milks, and other foods engineered in a lab. Over the last decade we've seen an explosion of "fake meat" and plant-based meat and dairy alternatives. Clearly, she understood the basic principles of capitalism.

Ellen White and the Seventh-day Adventist church laid the foundation for vegetarianism, but how did the anti-meat, high grain rhetoric take over our current guidelines? Let's take a moment and go back to the time period during World War II. During the war, the US wanted to ensure that our allies were properly fueled. Germany invaded Poland in 1939, and went on to invade the world. Almost every country was at war with the exception of the United States. Hunger became a major problem in Europe and Asia. The average caloric intake of Norwegians went from 2,500 calories before the war to 1,237 calories by the time the war was over.

The United States government responded by buying surplus food commodities, including wheat, corn, and sugar, and shipping them to allies. Farmers were given subsidies, which is money from the government, to continue to grow crops in large amounts to ensure adequate supply. The goal of subsidies was to keep the price of crops low and competitive. On December 7, 1941, the Japanese bombed the American Fleet in Pearl Harbor, Hawaii, prompting the United States to enter into the war. (43) Farmers were then called upon to produce *even more food*. They were no longer only fueling our allies, now they were also fueling our soldiers. Between 1940 and 1945, net cash income for farmers increased from 4.4 billion to 12.3 billion dollars. (13) After the war was over, the US government attempted to rescind all subsidies. This was not well received among farmers who were doing well with these new price controls. Some were removed, but many remain in place still today. After World War II, we had increased access to grains, corn, and wheat, but our nation was still eating meat, cheese, and butter, and drinking full fat milk.

In the late 1950's and early 1960's, Ancel Keys, mentioned earlier in this book, would come on to the nutrition scene. He would go on to become one of the most influential nutrition scientists of all time. Keys was among the first, if not *the* first, to hypothesize that heart disease was not an inevitable consequence of aging, but likely related to diet and lifestyle. He developed and directed the Seven Countries Study, and he concluded that dietary sources of saturated fat, notably meat and dairy, caused increased cardiovascular risk. He believed we needed to eat low-fat or no fat foods as well as dramatically reduce animal products and saturated fat. Keys was featured in *Time* magazine, and he was hailed as a leader in medicine and heart health.

Keys had an agenda, and that was to prove his theory that reducing animal products in the diet and reducing total cholesterol would prevent heart disease. **In order to prove his theory, he only reported data on the countries that fit his hypothesis.** It is curious to note that one of the places he visited to "prove" his hypothesis was the Greek isle of Crete. Also, he visited Crete during Lent, when most of the people abstain from eating dairy or meat. Keys did not include any countries in his report that would disprove his hypothesis. Some of these countries had the lowest rates of heart disease, and they consumed the most meat and dairy products.

Keys' "research" would go on to shape the Nutrition Guidelines of our nation. Shown by the graph below, our nation is experiencing an epidemic of obesity, diabetes, heart disease, and many other chronic ailments that threaten to bankrupt our health care system.

The graph below demonstrates what happened to our nation as we moved away from meat and saturated fat and began to consume more carbohydrates.

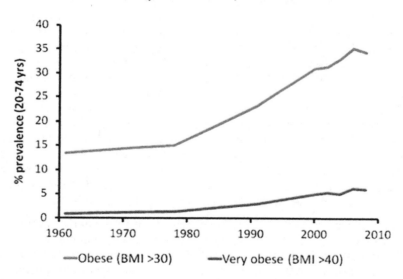

Obesity in the US, 1961-2009

CDC NHES and NHANES 1960-2008   USDA ERS loss-adjusted food disappearance

Picture Credit: "CDC - NCHS - National Center for Health Statistics." *Centers for Disease Control and Prevention*, Centers for Disease Control and Prevention, 7 Aug. 2020, www.cdc.gov/nchs/index.htm.

In 1967, Senators Rodger F. Kennedy and Joseph S. Clark took a field trip to the rural town of Cleveland, Mississippi. What they discovered there horrified the nation and launched a news special called *CBS Reports: Hunger in America*. They saw children suffering with severe malnutrition. At the time, this degree of starvation and malnutrition was thought to only exist in underdeveloped countries. Forms of extreme malnutrition, such as kwashiorkor and marasmus, were prevalent in poor, rural areas. (15) The public was horrified with images of bare cupboards and children with distended stomachs and bony arms and legs.

The government decided to create a committee to address hunger and undernutrition. The committee was called "The Select Committee on Nutrition and Human Needs," and it was headed by George McGovern. The bipartisan committee studied the problem of hunger and helped build momentum for a federal response. Senator Bob Dole, a Kansas Republican who served on the panel, said that due to its work and the field hearings it conducted, he could see that the problem was real and demanded a response. (19) This was the birth of the Food Stamps program, known today as the Supplemental Nutrition Assistance Program (SNAP). President Nixon and Congress acted on a bipartisan basis in 1971 to set national eligibility standards for food stamps based on household income and other financial resources and to ease barriers to enrollment that many of the poorest Americans faced. Congress took the program nationwide in 1974, mandating that every county participate, and then enacted the 1977 reforms. When the researchers returned to the same areas in the late 1970s, they found dramatic improvement, especially among children.

The Food Stamps program, started with the advocacy of the McGovern committee, was successful and the impacts were powerful and immediate. Children and families had access to very basic, yet adequate macronutrients for growth and development. (20)

What happened next is something many people can relate to. Did you have an opportunity to watch the movie *Kazaam*, released in 1996? I was thirteen when the movie came out, and it was agonizing to watch. Shaquille O'Neal, one of the top 10 greatest basketball players during my era, decided he would take up the role of "acting." It was abysmal. I remember being embarrassed for him. Many people are great athletes, actors, politicians, or doctors, and then they decide they will take on another role they have zero qualifications for. Terrible results can follow. Before we dive into that, we have to touch on the presidential campaign of the early 70's.

In 1971, Richard Nixon was facing reelection, and things in the United States were chaotic. The Vietnam War was in full swing and food prices were rising. Nixon needed to do something to show voters that he had a solution.

Nixon ended up hiring an agriculture expert, Earl Butz. Earl was an academic from Indiana, and Nixon was hoping Butz could help broker a deal with farmers to drive food costs down. He believed if food costs went down, he could earn the votes of the American public, because who doesn't like to save money? Butz had a plan that would have a dramatic, lasting impact on health as we knew it. He encouraged farmers to grow corn. Cows were fed corn, so they gained weight rapidly and became huge. Burgers were made bigger and french fries were no longer fried in tallow (animal fat) but were now fried in corn oil. Corn was everywhere! Flours, biscuits, and cereals began to be made with corn. Farmers became wealthy in a relatively short period of time due to the explosion of profit from growing corn. Unfortunately, there came a point where we had too much corn. What could we do with all this excess corn?

You may be able to guess what happened next. Butz flew to Japan where he had heard about a mass operation of turning corn into a cheap, sticky, sweet syrup which would be known as "high fructose corn syrup." This cheap, sweet goop was added to everything from pizza, to coleslaw, to meat, to cakes, bread, hot dogs, cereal, soup, and sauces. It made foods increasingly palatable and extended shelf life from several days to up to months at a time. And the cost of high fructose corn syrup was 2/3 less than sugar. In 1984 Coca Cola swapped its use of real sugar for high fructose corn syrup. Meanwhile, the general public had no idea that foods they had been eating for years were suddenly being injected with massive amounts of this stuff. (14)

Recall that the McGovern committee had a lasting impact on creating a system that could assist poor Americans in need of nutrition, but beginning in 1974, McGovern expanded the committee's scope to include national nutrition policy. (21) Now, the committee's focus was not just on helping poor Americans who were not eating enough; they would be tasked with helping Americans who were eating too much. (22, 23) Remember what happened with Shaq and *Kazaam*?

In 1977, enough consensus existed among epidemiologists that the McGovern committee, also called the U.S. Senate Select Committee on Nutrition and Human Need, decided to advocate dietary goals for an overall healthier diet for all Americans. In one year, the committee produced two editions of its *Dietary Goals for the United States*, the second containing a conciliatory statement about coronary heart disease and meat consumption. Critics have characterized the revision as a surrender to special interests. (16)

The committee subsequently entered a bitter policy battle with various interests, in particular the meat industry, over its dietary recommendations. During this period, the committee produced two editions of its *Dietary Goals for the United States*. The first, in February 1977, encouraged people to "decrease consumption of meat," (17) whereas the revised, more conciliatory edition, published 10 months later, urged Americans to "decrease consumption of animal fat, and choose meats...which will reduce saturated fat intake." (18)

In 1977 the committee, led by George McGovern, published the second edition, *Dietary Goals for the United States*, urging Americans to eat less high-fat red meat, eggs and dairy, and replace them with more calories from fruits, vegetables and especially carbohydrates. As you will see throughout this book, the "especially carbohydrates" part of this message would end up becoming particularly detrimental.

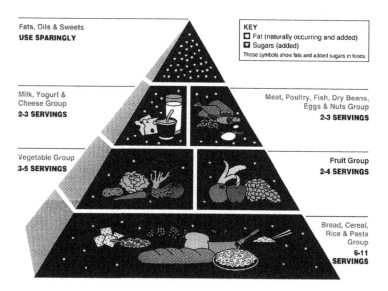

Picture: Original USDA Food Pyramid

By 1980 this governmental wisdom was officially put into print. The U.S. Department of Agriculture (USDA) issued its first dietary guidelines, and one of the primary messages was to avoid cholesterol and fat of all sorts. The National Institute of Health also recommended that all Americans over the age of two eat less fat and cholesterol to reduce risk of a heart attack. (24)

Now, you had the American people looking for alternatives to high-fat foods. At the same time, America as a country was dealing with a surplus of wheat, corn, and soybeans. We also had access to technology that could turn corn into high fructose corn syrup.

What a time to be a processed food manufacturer! Their highly processed, hyperpalatable foods might just be able to fit into this new "healthy whole grain, low fat agenda" set forth by the USDA. With the public looking for low-fat foods to stave off hunger and fulfill these new eating rules, several major food manufacturing companies employed scientists with the goal of finding the "bliss point" for their products. The bliss point is a term coined by American market researcher and psychophysicist, Howard Moskowitz. It is considered the amount of an ingredient, such as salt, sugar, or fat, which optimizes tastiness. It is literally someone's full time job to make chips and coffee creamer appeal to the human taste buds so much that they override the brain's ability to stop consuming. Some food manufacturing companies have used the bliss point ideals in their marketing. Most of us have heard, "Once you pop you can't stop" or "Bet you can't eat just one," in relation to snack foods.

Some people jokingly say things like, "I have a sweet tooth," or "I'm a choc-oholic," but these hyperpalatable foods may actually be addicting in the same way illicit substance are addicting. In an article titled, "The Addiction Potential of Hyperpalatable Foods," it is concluded that processed and re-fined foods "appear to have an abuse potential similar to addictive drugs like cocaine and alcohol." (25,26,27) The article concludes, "In summary, al-though highly processed foods differ from the traditional conceptualization of addictive drugs in some ways, such as the lack of intoxication, the degree of overlap is significant and compelling. In addition to neurobiological and behavioral similarities, hyperpalatable foods and addictive substances both trigger artificially high levels of reward, cause biological compensations that result in tolerance, and become linked with associated cues. Further, the components that increase the public health consequences of alcohol and nicotine are also present in the modern food environment, such as the ease of accessibility, increased social acceptability, heavy marketing, and lower cost of high calorie foods." (28) Many people have scoffed at the idea that you could *literally* be addicted to processed carbohydrates or sugar, but the evidence is compelling. You could be thrown in jail for providing your toddler with alcohol or tobacco, but you'll be deemed a "good parent" for giving a kiddo a highly processed, hyperpalatable, potentially addictive dessert.

Food manufacturers now had highly desirable, possibly addictive breads, snacks and cereals that could be produced for pennies and by the millions. The last hurdle to get over was how were they going to make sure that their products were viewed as a "part of this complete breakfast" or "part of an overall healthy meal."

The Academy of Nutrition is the governing board for all dietitians. Dieti-tians are supposed to take a firm stance on nutrition principles, and *all medical professionals* are under oath to first "do no harm." I became a dietitian in 2009, and I refused to be a member of the American Dietet-ic Association, now called the Academy of Nutrition, because I believed there was a huge conflict of interest with their cooperate sponsorship. Note: although it is encouraged and it comes with a $249 yearly fee, you are not required to be a member of the Academy of Nutrition to be a dietitian.

In 1995, a detailed report for the Academy's corporate sponsors was released. Not surprisingly, it included: McDonald's, PepsiCo, The Coca-Cola Company, Sara Lee, Abbott Nutrition, General Mills, Kellogg's, Mars, SoyJoy, Truvia, Unilever, and the Sugar Association. (30,31) Additionally, the Academy earns revenue from corporations by selling space at its booth during conventions, doing this for soft drinks and candy makers. In 2019, GlaxoSmithKline, a multinational pharmaceutical corporation, bought booth space at FNCE. FNCE is advertised as, "the world's largest gathering of food and nutrition experts." Doesn't it seem like a conflict of interest to have a company that sells diabetic drugs at an Academy of Nutrition convention?

What could sponsors like PepsiCo and General Mills possibly be buying? Certainly, dietitians would never walk into a patient room with a sugary cereal and a soda and declare it to be "healthy," right? This is correct. I have been practicing 11 years, and I have never seen something like that. What I have heard, repeatedly, and what you will see on blogs, Instagram accounts, and even medical advice columns, is something that is described so eloquently by Registered Dietitian and published author, Diana Rodgers. Diana recently published the book, *Sacred Cow,* where she advocates for meat for the health of humans and the planet. Diana describes exactly what PepsiCo, General Mills, and all the processed food companies bought when they agreed to sponsor the Academy of Nutrition:

"Many nutrition and medical experts counsel "moderation" and "finding balance." Although well intentioned, the advice is not only ineffective-it may even be injurious to people, as they blame themselves for "failure" instead of calling into question well-intentioned but terrible advice." (45)

Below is an example of a Continuing Education Credit (CEC) that I received on June 16, 2020, via email. (Please see graphic below.) Dietitians are required to take at least 75 CECs every 5 years to maintain their Registered Dietitian credentials. Depending on which state you practice in, you may have to fulfill additional requirements. For example, Oregon, where I practice, requires dietitians to obtain at least 15 CECs per year. At first glance, this CEC looks like it's about regenerative farming, which is a fantastic carbon-sequestering, planet benefiting process that we will discuss later in this book. If you look more closely, you will notice the CEC is sponsored by "General Mills' Bell Institute of Health and Nutrition." **And you may further notice "Learning Objective #3" in the flyer:** *"Participants will better understand the role packaged foods play in a sustainable diet and how dietitians can better educate their patients, clients and followers on this important topic."* ***This*** is what they are buying!

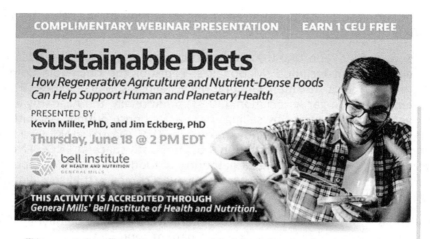

This presentation will provide an overview of the intersection of nutrient-dense foods and sustainability. We'll cover how General Mills is using regenerative agriculture practices to grow nutrient-dense food like oats and dairy more sustainably. We'll also cover what role packaged foods play in a sustainable diet and how dietitians can better educate their patients, clients and followers on this important topic.

Learning Objectives

1. Participants will gain knowledge in regenerative agriculture practices.
2. Participants will better understand the concept of nutrient-density and what it means to grow nutrient-dense foods from sustainable food systems.
3. Participants will better appreciate the role packaged foods play in a sustainable diet and how dietitians can better educate their patients, clients and followers on this important topic.

1 CEU FREE

Suggested CDR Learning Needs Codes: 2070, 8018, 4070, 4110
Suggested Performance Indicators: 8.1.1, 8.3.5, 12.1.1, 12.3.5
Level: 2

REGISTER NOW

It breaks my heart when I see dietitians posting blogs and making Instagram posts about "all foods in moderation," while they show pictures of themselves and their families eating donuts or slamming sodas. While this idea of "all foods can fit" and "balance" sounds nice, moderation is an abstract concept at best, and a dangerous gateway to addiction at worst. Now that you've had an opportunity to learn about neurotransmitters, that statement may not sound so extreme. Sugar, processed carbohydrates, and seed oils can alter brain activity and cause inflammation. Every individual who provided their testimony, referenced a *genuine desire* to follow the nutrition guidelines for health. As you read through the testimonies, you will see stories of men and women who struggled with food addiction, obesity, anxiety, and depression for years at the hands of this terrible advice. Some of these individuals were completely convinced that there was something fundamentally wrong with them versus something fundamentally wrong with our recommendations.

When you combine the fact that humans cannot moderate processed carbohydrates well, if at all, due to the reasons described above, as well as the inconvenient truth that no one knows what exactly defines "in moderation," you have the makings of a massive profit for processed food companies and a nation that is sick, fat, and dying of highly preventable, chronic diseases. As we have discussed throughout this book, patients are often told to eat "sweets in moderation," and "fat in moderation," and to "exercise in moderation." This advice is useless. When people fail because eating carbohydrates goes against human physiology, the patient is blamed for being "lazy" or "gluttonous."

Is it possible that processed food companies purchased the idea of moderation being taught by nutrition experts? Some of these companies even went above and beyond that by adding whole wheat flour to their processed foods to further encourage nutrition experts to recommend them. The whole wheat flour causes blood sugar surges similar or worse, in some cases, than white flour. Adding whole wheat flour allowed food manufacturers' granola bars and cereals to fit into the bottom of the pyramid and be part of a "balanced diet."

Food manufacturers began to advertise that their products could be part of the "Healthy Whole Grain" food pyramid section. Corn, wheat, and oats soaked in sugar or high fructose corn syrup were now "part of a complete breakfast." At the same time, largely thanks to the groundwork of Ellen White and incomplete reporting from Ancel Keys, animal proteins and fat were considered dangerous for health and to be avoided.

If you grew up in the 1990's, you likely remember hearing about when everything was "low fat" and "nonfat." Fat free became all the rage. There was low-fat yogurt, cheese, salad dressing, cereal, bread, meat dishes, beverages, desserts, etc. I remember as a young dietitian thinking it was interesting that people wouldn't read ingredients, but simply focus on calories and grams of fat. It didn't matter if a cereal was made of wheat flour, sugar and preservatives. By golly, if it only had 2 grams of fat per serving it much be good for you! Low fat equated health in the minds of many Americans. Of course, when fat was initially removed from processed food items, the food tasted terrible. Food processers realized very quickly that removing fat from processed food items made them taste like cardboard. What did they do? What is cheap and easy to add, and can improve the taste of our food? Sugar, or more specifically during this time period, high fructose corn syrup.

These guidelines became so powerful and so fundamentally ingrained in dietetics and medicine, that even a major retraction issued in 2014, stating there was no association between dietary cholesterol and fat and heart disease, cancer, and diabetes, did not cause the guidelines to change. (9,10,11)

What's perhaps even more astounding is that it was discovered in 2016 that Harvard Scientists were paid to blame dietary fat for heart disease when the true culprit was sugar. In the 1960's, when Americans were attempting to figure out which foods could contribute to heart disease, two prominent nutritionists from Harvard, Fredrick J. Stare and D. Mark Hegsted, worked closely with a trade group called the Sugar Research Foundation. The Sugar Research Foundation was concerned that if Americans discovered how detrimental sugar was to heart health, they would see a decrease in profits. They paid the current equivalent of $48,000 to Stare and Hegsted to downplay sugar's role in heart disease and use cherry-picked data to put the blame on fat and saturated fat. This "research" was published in two prominent journals at the time. In the 1960's, it didn't have to be disclosed where funding for published research was coming from, so there was no way for the public to know that The Sugar Research Foundation was funding the studies that insisted, "It's not sugar, it's fat." (12)

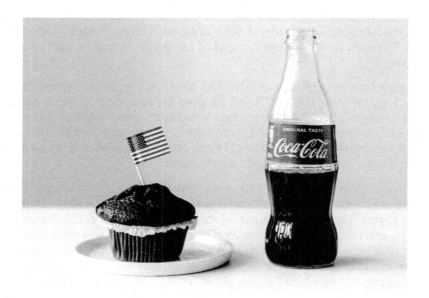

If you research the Academy of Nutrition's official stance on vegetarian diets, you will see the work of three experts, Vesanto Melina, Winston J. Craig, and Susan Levin. All of these "experts" claimed there was no conflict of interest when writing their official statement, which states vegetarian diets are adequate and healthy for all humans across the lifecycle. Unfortunately, in truth all of these individuals are either ideological vegetarians or vegans, or they have a vested financial interest in official acceptance of this diet. (7)

That sounds like a potential conflict of interest to me. Vesanto Melina, a Canadian dietitian, describes herself as "a consultant for individuals who would like to fine tune their plant-based diets," and has authored a dozen books on vegan and vegetarian diets. I find it particularly troubling that one of her books talks about how to raise children without meat. Winston J. Craig is a professor of nutrition at Andrews University, which is a Seventh-day Adventist institution. The mission of this institution states they are to, "prepare dietetic and nutrition professionals for service in the church, society, and the world and to influence the community-at large to affirm the Seventh-day Adventist lifestyle, including vegetarian diet." Not surprisingly, Mr. Craig is also the author of several vegetarian books and research papers. Finally, let's talk about Susan Levin. She is currently the director of nutrition education for the Physicians Committee for Responsible Medicine. She is a vegan activist, and as a dietitian, I have personally come across her continuing education courses for dietic professionals. One such course is called *Eating Vegan Through the Lifecycle*. This means she supports children as well as the elderly following a diet void of all animal products. She also has published a continuing education course called, *Meat as a Risk Factor for Diabetes*. As you saw in our chapter on diabetes, following a high-meat, high-fat diet can reverse diabetes in as little as nine days. Ignoring the clinical trials and putting out this type of rhetoric purely for profit appears to me to be unethical.

To recap, the guidelines were highly influenced by the vegetarian visions of Ellen White, who thought meat made you horny, and by her creation of "medical evangelism" through the Seventh-day Adventist Church. World War II saw farmers making money and getting subsidies, some of which are still in place today. In the late 60's people became aware of food insecurity and malnutrition in the United States, which led to the McGovern committee. This committee was largely successful in helping alleviate malnutrition but was tasked with tackling obesity in America. After the influence of Ancel Keys and the overwhelming amount of corn, wheat, and high fructose corn syrup available and marketed the United States, there was a dramatic shift in how Americans ate, and obesity and chronic diseases increased exponentially.

The McGovern committee would go on to recommend Americans consume lots of grains and less meat and fat. The "less meat and fat" ideals would continue to be propagated by vegans and vegetarians who made up the Academy of Nutrition's governing board in the 1980's. Food manufacturers would get in bed with the Academy of Nutrition in exchange for telling patients to, "only consume their products in moderation," fully knowing their products had been designed to override the brain's ability to moderate them. We saw a public admission that Harvard nutritionists were paid to throw fat under the bus instead of sugar, and more evidence than ever that saturated fat, in the absence of high blood sugar, has zero relation to heart disease and other chronic diseases.

What do we do? Unfortunately, many people believe it is time to return to a plant-based diet. While the Academy's position on this way of eating says it can be optimal for humans at any age, it is my hope you take the information provided in my book seriously. It is my life story and life's work to make a case that while some plants can absolutely fit into many people's diets, a diet that *is mostly plants (or plant-based)*, is a disaster for human health and for the planet.

Most companies who are urging people to "go vegan" or "go plant-based" have millions of dollars invested in fake meat products. James Cameron, best known for producing movies such as *Titanic, Aliens*, and *Terminator*, co-produced the vegan documentary, *Game Changers*, which advocates a vegan diet. (32,33) He is in a million-dollar business venture with business partner and fellow heavyweight filmmaker, Peter Jackson, to produce plant-based meat, cheese, and dairy products. As you have seen in this book, animal products are dense in highly absorbable protein, vitamins, minerals, collagen, and essential fat. There is a reason that zero cultures and tribes throughout history have been vegan.

As time goes on and the public continues to see the success of ketogenetic, low-carbohydrate, high-meat diets, expect a lot more research papers to come forward and suggest, very carefully, in a very businesslike way, basically, Oops! *Our bad. Meat isn't the problem.* In 2019, the dietary guideline recommendations from the Nutrition Recommendation Consortium were released. They noted that we do not have the evidence to support encouraging Americans to eat less red meat. (2) That sounds a lot more professional than, *Holy crap, if people were eating more red meat and less carbohydrates over the last 30 years, instead of following our recommendations, we could have potentially prevented thousands of cases of diabetes and heart disease.*

You don't need to wait for the guidelines to change. If you are reading this book, it's my hope that you have an open mind, common sense, and critical thinking skills.

What are you waiting for?

Stacy Chrzanowski

Instagram: @healthy.carnivore.stacy

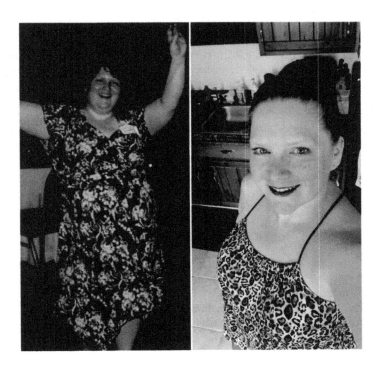

My name is Stacy Czarnowski. I am 44 years old and am the healthiest I have been in my life, thanks to switching to a zero carb/carnivore way of eating. I'm a Registered Nurse in a busy Emergency Department, and during the COVID-19 crisis I also worked in our ICU to assist with the increased demands of such a high number of critically ill patients. I'm grateful my improved health allowed me to stay strong during that trying time. I have lived most of my life with Hypothyroidism, which was diagnosed when I was 8 years old. I didn't really understand it well until about 5 years ago. I also developed Polycystic Ovary Syndrome (PCOS) as a young teen, and I suffered through painful menstrual cycles, missed periods, and ovarian cysts, causing me to have to have surgery. I have lived with cycles of depression and anxiety, requiring therapy and sometimes medication. I now acknowledge that I suffered from bulimia and binge eating disorder, and I was placed on medication to control my blood pressure at the age of 26.

My weight has been a struggle for as long as I can remember, and I understand now that so many of my ailments could have been prevented or treated with appropriate nutrition and the avoidance of foods that I now know are inflammatory to me. I can vividly remember being sent to school in the 3rd grade with a 1/2 sandwich on light bread, fat-free yogurt and carrot sticks, because my parents were worried about my weight. I was cold and tired and lacked energy and still remember feeling like I was in a fog. I was diagnosed that year with Hypothyroidism. Taking Synthroid helped, but it didn't really fix anything. My parents just followed the doctor's orders and thought they were doing all they could. Back then, nutrition guidelines were so entrenched in the low fat, low sodium movement, that they wouldn't have even known there was another way. I was "gifted" a membership to Weight Watchers by my grandparents when I was in the 8th grade, and my grandmother came to meetings with my mother and I to pay the bill. It worked for a few years, and I have gravitated back to their methods many times over the years. Unfortunately, this is also where the binge eating and laxative use started. I would feel so restricted that I would binge on cookies or ice cream and then take laxatives to be sure I could still show weight loss when we went to meetings. I went back and forth between counting calories and bulimia through high school and then lost all control when I found myself in an abusive relationship. I gained 100lbs in my first year living with this person, and I struggled to lose that weight for over 24 years.

Over the years, I tried many different methods to try and lose weight, some smarter than others, but always ended up going back to binging and gaining the weight back. I tried Atkins in my late 20's and had success for about a year. I realize now that I didn't succeed back then because I still needed to change my mindset, and I just wasn't ready. I first learned about the possibility of Zero Carb when I came across a link to Kelly Williams Hogan's blog, My Zero Carb Life, in 2015. Kelly detailed her incredible story of healing after removing plants from her diet and I was intrigued, not enough to try it yet, but intrigued. I gravitated into keto and had success but it was never long term. I found I would still have cravings and "cheat" and the binge eating was still lurking. I did manage to wean myself off antidepressant medication during this time, but I was still struggling with anxiety and depression. In 2018, I became aware of zero carb or carnivore when I saw Jordan Peterson and Dr. Shawn Baker each interviewed on The Joe Rogan Experience. That really got me thinking. In July of 2018, I went carnivore for 5 weeks and felt incredible, then we went on vacation and I ate everything in sight and threw myself into a tailspin.

Finally, in February of 2019 I was fed up again with how miserable I was feeling and decided to start keto again. After a week I was having full sugar ice cream after a tough overnight shift and having to start over, again. I decided to do more research about cutting out all plants, artificial sweeteners and seed oils, and just finally making a change. I WAS READY.

March 13th, 2019 was the first day of the rest of my life. I cooked myself a beautiful ribeye steak and have not looked back. Over the next several weeks my body dumped oxalates, I suffered eczema flare ups and joint pain and GI upset but that all passed relatively quickly and I made it to the other side. I realized that I felt so good and full of energy and free from pain that sugary foods no longer tempted me. I didn't want to go back to feeling the way I did before. I found myself eating a large meal 1 or 2 times per day and then not eating in between. I think this helped my binge eating because I was able to give myself permission to eat a large, decadent, rich and buttery steak and feel truly satisfied and then I just wouldn't eat again until I was hungry. I realized that I am allowed to eat wonderful foods that make me feel happy and healthy and I don't like how I feel if I eat "cheats". I used artificial sweetener one afternoon and my stomach was in so much pain afterward. I ate a few carrots mixed into chicken meatballs and had an eczema flare up the next day. Neither of those things is worth trying again. At least not now.

In addition to my better sleep, energy, moods, digestion, and skin, (I even tan in the sun and don't burn like a lobster!) I have lost weight, reduced my requirement for Synthroid, weaned off blood pressure meds, and simply feel like a whole new person.

My hope is that my story will help to inspire someone else to make smarter choices for themselves, take their health into their own hands and look to alternative sources for their information. As a nurse, I see so many people every day who would benefit immensely from making even a few changes to how they eat. I try to council where I can but am bound by the rules of my employer. I share my own story with these people as well and hope it steers them in a new direction.

Robert Sikes

(Creator of the Keto Brick)
Instagram: @liveSavage and @ketobrick
Website: https://www.ketobrick.com/

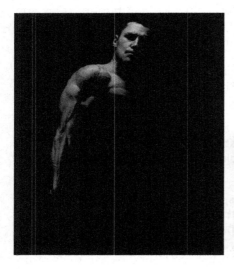
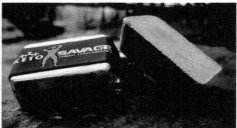

Robert Orion Sikes is a lifetime natural, competitive bodybuilder. He started training as a junior in high school weighing a whopping 115 pounds. In the beginning, he followed traditional, "bro-dieting" wisdom which consisted of eating 6 or 7 meals a day filled with carbohydrates and very high protein. This nutritional protocol led to a downward spiral of health issues and disordered eating.

After his third bodybuilding competition, Robert decided to try something new and began experimenting with a high-fat, strict ketogenic approach to bodybuilding. He formulated his own approach to contest prep nutrition leveraging keto and earned his pro-status with bodybuilding in 2017. He has since dedicated his life to learning and teaching others the benefits of following a well formulated, ketogenic lifestyle. The lessons learned led to his creation of the Keto Brick, a 1,000 calorie, ketogenic performance meal. The Brick was never meant to be a product sold to the public. Robert just created it for his own personal use during his competition prep. However, after featuring it on a YouTube video, he received a ton of interest around the Brick and decided to jump in with both feet to make it into a viable business. After countless late nights and a never-ending grind, the business took off and has since become a wild success!

Robert now works alongside his wife, Crystal, and their amazing team to continually create content and Bricks, and add a ton of value within this community. His mission is, and will continue to be, empowering others to believe in themselves and truly tap into their full potential by optimizing their body and mind.

Chapter 7:

Plants vs Animals

Before we get into the meat of this chapter, pun intended, I want to take a minute to acknowledge that the human diet is an emotionally charged topic. People will defend their dietary habits similarly to how they defend their religious beliefs. I've had a few people tell me that they would *never* change how they ate, even if it meant their current diet would lead to a decline in their health or an early death. If you or someone you know falls into this category, there is likely very little I can do to change your mind. If you are open to exploring a different approach, I can promise you that the potential restoration of your physical and mental health could make every aspect of your life better. When you feel better, it's much easier to live a life that has a positive impact on the people around you and our planet as a whole. Intriguing, isn't it? So, without further ado, let's dive in.

As I became more interested in human evolution, and I took the time to dig into what an optimal diet for humans really looks like, I arrived at two conclusions. The first conclusion is that we have our macronutrient ratios backwards. Our current nutrition guidelines recommend 50-60% carbohydrates, 30-35% fat, and approximately 15% protein. (5) As we've continued to consume more plants, carbohydrates, and seed oils while concurrently reducing our saturated animal fat and meat intake, the rate of chronic disease, including autoimmune conditions, have skyrocketed.

The second conclusion we will explore is that a relatively large percentage of the population believes meat is not only bad for your health but is bad for the planet. In their efforts to protect their health, their family's health, and the condition of the planet, many individuals have given up eating meat. Some individuals believe that abstaining from all animal products is the best way to restore human health and combat climate change. Often, these beliefs are based on emotionally charged statements that ignore human physiology and our role in the ecosystem. It's not uncommon to hear things like, "Meat is murder," or "If you eat meat, you're causing suffering," and "Humans don't need meat to survive." Hopefully, by this point in the book, you have begun to understand and appreciate the role animal products have in providing absorbable nutrition for our bodies and brains. I mentioned Diana Rodgers' book, *Sacred Cow*, earlier, which specifically addresses animal agriculture and meats' impact on the planet. For an incredibly detailed discussion on regenerative agriculture and how it protects the planet, I recommend investing in her book.

In this chapter, we will discuss several points to consider when you are deciding what types of food to put into your body. We will begin with reviewing what foods provide the most nutrient-dense, bioavailable nutrition for the human body. We will answer the question, *What foods are humans able to extract the most nutrition from?* Next, we will discuss what foods the human body and brain crave and desire consistently. This ties into sustainability because intuitively, it makes sense that most people are not going to follow a way of eating for a long period of time if the food isn't delicious, palatable, and satiating. Finally, we will discuss how the foods we eat affect the planet. Is eating a vegan or vegetarian diet truly better for planet?

Bioavailability

The first point we will discuss is bioavailability. Recall that this term simply means how much nutrition your body can actually use from any individual food. *Bioavailability is species specific, meaning some animals can get all the nutrition they need from certain substances like plants, while some species simply cannot.*

Let's begin with the simple fact that you are a human. Ideally, the way you fuel your body should align with human physiology. In their zeal to demonize animal products, some individuals forget that humans, like any other species, have a natural diet that is *designed for their specific physiological makeup.* Animals like cows, sheep, or gorillas have a very different physiological make-up than humans. These animals' anatomy contributes to their ability to effectively digest and extract nutrition from plant foods.

Humans' physiological make up contributes to an ineffective ability to digest and extract nutrition from plant foods. As a dietitian, I have spoken with many people who are convinced that eating large quantities of plants is necessary for good health. Throughout my dietetics career, it has been routinely emphasized to me that all plant foods are healthy, anti-inflammatory, and nourishing. In reality, many plant foods may not be well digested or well absorbed by the human body. In certain cases, these foods may contribute to inflammation, disease, and autoimmune disorders.

Some species, like the gorilla in the picture below, have a physiological design and function which is very different from humans. Often, vegans and vegetarians point to the gorilla as an example of how any living species should be able to eat a plant-based diet and experience vibrant health and great strength. It is true that gorillas are incredibly strong. They can lift over 10 times their body weight! Gorillas spend quite a bit of time chewing on leaves, bark, and other vegetation to obtain the 40 pounds of plant material they consume a day. Gorillas have a big belly which is necessary because the size of their colon is both longer and larger than a human's so they can ferment the plant fibers they eat. This fermentation results in the production of short chain fatty acids which are used as their main source of their energy. Gorillas are eating 40 pounds of carbohydrate-based plant matter, but their ability to ferment these plants in their guts allows *them to be running off fat.* **Humans do not have this ability.**

When humans eat plant materials, we break down and absorb the starches which are either used for energy or go directly into glycogen (carbohydrate)

WHY WE CAN'T

EAT LIKE COWS

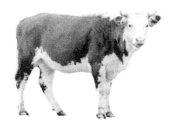

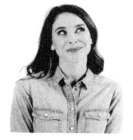

CATTLE DIGESTION

4 compartments in stomach

Food is fermented in gut, is regurgitated and chewed again

Fermentation turns plant matter into nutrients

16 hours a day spent eating

HUMAN DIGESTION

1 compartment in stomach

Food is chewed only once and then broken down by enzymes

Cannot turn plant matter into nutrients, need bioavaliable nutrients

<2 hours a day spent eating

or fat storage. We are not able to burn, utilize, or run-on fat for fuel when we take in large doses of carbohydrates. The insulin response that occurs after eating a high-carbohydrate plant-based meal, such as beans, rice, and vegetables, will prevent fatty acid oxidation from occurring. When you eat starchy, carbohydrate rich plant foods plants, you suppress your body's ability to burn fat due to an insulin response. This is the opposite of what most people need when they are attempting to lose weight or simply desire consistent energy. When humans eat cellulose, which is fiber from plants, it cannot be broken down by enzymes. Only a small part of the cellulose will be broken down by our gut microbes in the large intestine. When you consume large amounts of plant foods, you will likely experience a solid amount of bloating and gas from the fermentation that occurs in the colon. Due to an insulin response from starch and sugars, you may feel the need to eat an hour or so later even if you consumed quite a few calories in your high-carbohydrate, plant-based meal.

WHY WE CAN'T

EAT LIKE GORILLAS

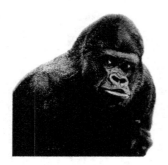

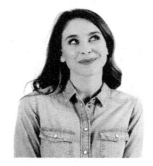

GORILLA DIGESTION

Colon 3x the size of small intestine

Large colon is suitable for breaking down fiborous plants

Big belly is necessary for large colon

Eats 18kg (40lb) of food a day

HUMAN DIGESTION

Colon 1/2 the size of small intestine

Large small intenstine suitable for dense, smaller volume foods

Big belly caused by visceral fat

Less volume of food required

Antinutrients

Could eating plants be dangerous to your health? The mere thought of beans, broccoli, or spinach causing harm in the human body goes against everything we are taught about nutrition. From a young age, most of us are told to, "Eat your vegetables," and certainly there is a movement at this current juncture in history for humans to embrace a plant-based diet. The idea that eating lots of rice, potatoes, or quinoa could potentially be a bad idea due to the amount of concentrated starch in these plants makes sense, but what about high fiber, low calorie vegetables like spinach, swiss chard, or tomatoes?

Some individuals find they tolerate small amounts of plant foods including certain vegetables and even some grains. For many people, however, the majority of grains and many plant foods have more potential downsides than upsides.

WHAT ARE ANTINUTRIENTS?

LECTINS

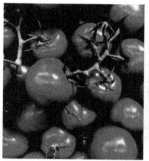

Bind to minerals + stops
their absorption

Damages the gut wall

**Wheat, soybeans, beans,
peanuts + tomatoes**

OXALATE

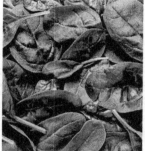

Bind to minerals + stops
their absorption

Form 80% of kidney stones

**Spinach, rhubarb, rice
bran, almonds + wheat**

PHYTATE

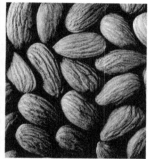

Bind to minerals + stops
their absorption

Has some health benefits

**Almonds, beans, nuts,
corn, lentils + wheat**

As we discussed briefly in our chapter on sarcopenia, every living organism in nature, including all plants and animals, has the desire to survive. In order to reproduce and continue its lineage, ending up as lunch for a hungry predator is not on any plant or animal's "To Do" list.

Unlike animals, plants cannot run away if a predator attempts to eat them. They are literally rooted into the ground. Throughout evolution, plants developed powerful defense mechanisms to prevent animals, birds, and humans from eating them. Many plants are incredibly bitter tasting, and some plants can actually kill you if you don't prepare them properly. For example, the cassava root, otherwise known as yuca, is a staple food for over half a billion people. Due to its high content of cyanide, it is one of the most drought-resistant, pest-resistant sources of carbohydrates in the tropics. Cassava, especially bitter cassava, must be processed before consumption, or the individual consuming the cassava could die of cyanide poisoning.

Plants contain several compounds called antinutrients that can be potentially dangerous to human health. Antinutrients are defined as compounds in plants that interfere with the human body's ability to absorb minerals. Antinutrients include: saponins, phytic acid (phytates), gluten, tannins, oxalates, lectins, polyphenols, flavonoids, trypsin inhibiters, isoflavones, solanine, and chaconine12. Below, I'll briefly break down four of the most common antinutrients and their effects on human health.

Phytic Acid, or Phytates

Phytic acid is found in all grains, seeds, beans and nuts. Phytic acid impairs the absorption of iron, zinc, magnesium, copper, and calcium and may promote mineral deficiencies. It is not unusual for vegans or vegetarians to be iron deficient due to a diet high in grains and beans. (2) Endurance athletes consuming high amounts of carbohydrates in the form of grains may also be deficient in iron, calcium, or magnesium due to the effects of the high phytate content in plant foods. Phytates also inhibit the digestive enzymes pepsin, trypsin and amylase. Amylase is required for the breakdown of starch, while trypsin and pepsin are involved in the breakdown of protein. By inhibiting the breakdown of starch and protein, it is possible that consuming high amounts of phytic acid in your diet will prevent your body from absorbing the amino acids, vitamins, and minerals in the foods you are eating.

What happens when an elderly person replaces steak with beans, which are high in phytic acid, or chows down on a peanut butter sandwich, also high in phytic acid, every day instead of eating a chicken thigh or omelet? Could phytates be contributing to osteoporosis and other bone degrading diseases in the elderly? One study showed a remarkable improvement in bone density when rats were fed phytase, which is an enzyme supplement designed to break down and reduce the mineral robbing effects of phytate. (1) Phytase is not an enzyme that naturally occurs in the human body. If someone chooses to include foods high in phytic acid in their diet, it makes sense to prepare them in a way that reduces the phytate content. This can be accomplished through preparation methods including soaking, sprouting, or cooking.

Lectins

Lectins occur across the plant and animal kingdom, yet the lectins from plants tend to have detrimental health implications for humans. Humans do not process lectins from plants well. To understand how damaging lectins can be to the human body, it's important to know a little bit about the gastrointestinal tract.

Most of the organisms of the gastrointestinal microbiome can be found on the surface of the gut atop a protective layer of mucus. Under this layer, there is a single layer of cells known as the gastrointestinal epithelium. This layer of cells which align the stomach and intestines are extremely important in allowing good substances into the bloodstream and keeping harmful substances out of the blood stream. A mucus layer protects the cells from harmful pathogens such as bacteria and viruses. (3) Lectins are proteins that can cause trouble in the digestive system by sticking to the intestinal wall. (2) When food moves through the digestive system, it collides with the GI tract and can potentially cause small traumas. This is not usually an issue as the cells along the GI tract quickly repair any damage that occurs. Unfortunately, lectins can prevent the GI tract from repairing. This means the damage that normally wouldn't be a big deal because it can be repaired quickly, may become a very big deal because the presence of lectins prevents healing. Over time, an unrepaired, damaged gut ends up irritated and inflamed. If you eat a lot of lectins, there is a potential for the continued damage in your gut to cause holes in the GI lining. This causes contents of the gut to leak into the blood stream. This condition, known as "Leaky Gut Syndrome," can cause an array of symptoms, including fatigue, joint pain, constipation, diarrhea, and difficulty concentrating.

There is a lectin found in potatoes called "solanum tuberosum agglutinin" which activates the cells of the immune system. This activation has been known to release histamines which can cause swelling, itching, and hives. (4) Studies of multiple foods including soybeans, lentils, wheat germ, and kidney beans demonstrated that lectins from these foods could bind to white blood cells. Once bound, the white blood cells release a signal stating, *We have a foreign invader! Something is wrong!* and they release inflammatory cytokines.

Releasing inflammatory cytokines is *really important* when something is *actually wrong.* For example, if you have a bacterial infection, you want to release some inflammatory cytokines and cause inflammation in your body to bring resources to fight the infection. If there is no real threat, releasing inflammatory cytokines causes unnecessary inflammation and swelling throughout the body. In the case of lectins, this is like the fire alarm going off in the office and everyone rushing outside and standing in the rain. The fire department is called, you're soaked and miserable, and you find out Bob put the popcorn in the microwave, set it for 8 minutes, and walked away. It's a false alarm, but the damage is done. It's important to note that individual tolerance with lectins *varies widely.* Some people are able to eat foods with lectins and experience few side effects, while some individuals can eat one food with a lectin protein and experience debilitating, autoimmune symptoms.

The most common sources of lectins include grains, legumes, and nightshades. Nightshades include tomatoes, white potatoes, eggplant, bell peppers, chili peppers, tobacco, and goji berries. Common symptoms of lectin sensitivity include inflammation, migraines, stomach issues, acne or joint pain after eating a lectin-rich meal. The lectins in nightshades are a common autoimmune trigger and can cause sensitivities in many people. For individuals who are lecithin sensitive, removal of these vegetables from the diet often results in significant improvements in joint pain, arthritis, and other autoimmune symptoms.

Oxalates

Oxalates are produced in very small quantities as a waste product of human metabolism. Oxalates are shaped like needles or crystals (see image below) and when ingested in large enough quantities, they can damage the human body. Foods very high in oxalates include spinach, swiss chard, rhubarb, beans, blackberries, peanuts, almonds, turmeric, beets, and potatoes. The symptoms of oxalate accumulation include pain, nephrolithiasis, and neurological symptoms. While consuming foods high in oxalates may not initially cause symptoms, oxalate crystals can build up in the tissues of the body over time. There is currently research being done which is linking years of oxalate buildup to conditions such vulvodynia (vulvar pain), fibromyalgia pain, and leaky gut syndrome.

Oxalate crystals under a microscope:

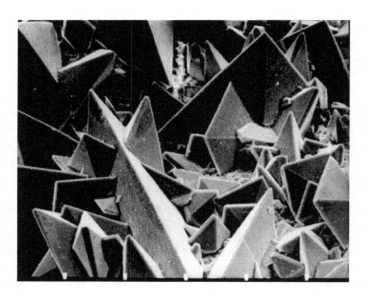

Humans produce 10-30 mg of oxalates per day through the glyoxylate pathway and through protein breakdown. If you make a "healthy" green smoothie with spinach, swiss chard, almonds, and turmeric powder, you could easily end up with 100-200 times the amount of oxalates your body naturally produces daily. While this may not seem like a big deal, there have been several documented cases of people dying by consuming as little as 5,000 mg of oxalates. (53, 54, 55) You could reach this amount by taking large doses of turmeric or drinking several highly concentrated spinach smoothies. The most common medical condition caused by consuming foods high in oxalates is kidney stones. A study conducted by The American Journal of Renal (Kidney) Physiology concluded, "To limit calcium oxalate stone growth (kidney stones) we advocate that patients avoid oxalate rich foods." (52)

Consuming microscopic needles, or foods high in oxalates, in large quantities would appear to not be ideal for the general population, but research shows it could be detrimental for individuals with certain conditions. In 2011, a study found that children with autism displayed *three times the normal level of oxalates in their blood stream and two and half times the normal levels of oxalates in their urine. (51)* The researchers concluded, "Whether this is a result of impaired renal (kidney) excretion, extensive intestinal absorption, or both, or whether oxalates may cross the blood-brain barrier and disturb central nervous system function in autistic children remains unclear." Basically, they don't know if it's because the kidneys aren't getting rid of the oxalates, the intestinal tract is absorbing all the oxalates, or the oxalates are crossing the blood-brain barrier in children with autism. What they do know is that children with autism are ending up with excessive levels of oxalates in their bloodstream and urine.

The best way to reduce oxalates in the body is to reduce or eliminate them from the diet.

Gluten

After Dr. William Davis released his book, *Wheat Belly*, many people started thinking twice about eating foods with gluten. Gluten is defined as a family of storage proteins present in cereal grains, especially wheat, that is responsible for the elastic texture of dough. (42) It's well documented that gluten can cause serious, potentially life-threatening issues in individuals with celiac disease. (43) Apart from individuals with diagnosed celiac disease, can eating foods with gluten, or other components in wheat, cause harm? There have been several studies that indicate that gluten itself can cause inflammation in individuals with non-celiac gluten sensitivity. (44,45,46) Many individuals without celiac disease who are dealing with chronic autoimmune symptoms, report reduction of inflammation, rashes, fatigue, bloating, and brain fog when completely removing all gluten containing foods from their diets. Some researchers hypothesize it is not the gluten but agglutinin, a part of the wheat germ, that triggers systemic inflammation in susceptible individuals. (47,48) Finally, there have been additional studies that show that amylase trypsin inhibitors, present in wheat, may play a role in causing allergies, asthma, irritable bowel syndrome, and arthritis. (49,50) Whether it's gluten, agglutinin, or amylase trypsin inhibitors, it's clear that for some individuals, consuming foods with these antinutrients can have negative health consequences and should be minimized or avoided.

Bioavailability

When it comes to the bioavailability of nutrition, remember that the human body is like a supercomputer; it needs the correct input to give the correct output. Look at the illustration below for an example to illustrate bioavailability. It does your body no good if a food contains 2.6 mg of your daily iron needs, but your body can only absorb and utilize less than 1.7% of the iron in that food. Spinach is a good example of a food that has would very poor bioavailability for the mineral iron. Recall our earlier analogy. It would be like if I wrote you a check for $1,000, but you find out I only have 17 dollars in my bank account. Just like it doesn't matter how much the check is written for if you can't access the funds, it doesn't matter how much of a particular micronutrient a certain food contains if the human body can't absorb and use it. Unlike spinach, beef has a 20% absorption rate for iron. This food is considered to have good bioavailability. **It's imperative that we note that nutrition labels *do not show bioavailability*.** I believe this has caused massive confusion in the debate over whether plants or animals are best for human health.

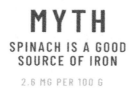

MYTH

SPINACH IS A GOOD
SOURCE OF IRON

2.6 MG PER 100 G

FACT

BEEF IS A BETTER
SOURCE OF IRON

2.5 MG PER 100 G

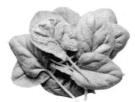

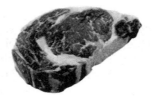

1.7%
ABSORPTION RATE

0.044 MG
NET TOTAL

20%
ABSORPTION RATE

0.5 MG
NET TOTAL

When it comes to providing the most bioavailable nutrition for the human body, animal products, especially ruminant muscle tissue, fat, and organs, win by a landslide. Despite the hopeful visions of Ellen White, plant foods do not contain vitamin B12. Some plant-based nutritionists have insisted that you can get adequate B12 from algae, but studies show this is not the case. In fact, the B12 analogues in algae *increase* the human bodies need for real, animal based B12. (6) Not surprisingly, vitamin B12 is one of the most prevalent deficiencies in the vegetarian and vegan population. A full 60% of adult vegans and 40% of adult vegetarians have been found to be deficient in B12. (7,8) Vitamin B12 deficiency can cause irreversible consequences for children including delayed cognitive development, irreversible nerve damage, and failure to thrive. Studies are also showing there is a link to Alzheimer's disease and inadequate intake of the B12 vitamin.

Recall from our chapter on sarcopenia that the elderly population doesn't meet the current bare minimum requirement for protein intake. B12 is only found in the animal kingdom and is specifically found in meat and dairy. A recent study found that low levels of B12 (under 250 mol/L) are associated with Alzheimer's disease, vascular dementia, and Parkinson's disease. (58) This demonstrates the importance of ensuring adequate levels of B12 to preserve and maintain brain function, especially as we age. In my experience working in acute care for many years, I witnessed many seniors eating very small (if any) portions of protein, and their labs often indicated B12 deficiency. Typically, seniors fill up on nutrient poor, starchy foods. A standard hospital breakfast for a senior consists of french toast with syrup, apple slices, orange juice, and coffee. A standard hospital lunch or dinner for a senior consists of a 2-3-ounce portions of turkey, mashed potatoes with margarine, a roll, apple juice, and one or two chocolate chip cookies.

Many seniors are being told they need to "reduce meat" to be healthy. To many people this means simply dropping the meat and adding more carbohydrates. I often see patients eliminating the turkey, eggs, or meatloaf from the breakfast or dinner meal and having an extra roll, pastry, or cookie. As we discussed in our chapter on diabetes, consuming excessive carbohydrates in the form of bread, fruit, or sugar overtime can cause insulin resistance and diabetes.

One of the most popular diabetic prescription drugs is metformin. Metformin is a used for lowering blood glucose concentrations in patients with type 2 diabetes, particularly in those overweight and obese as well as those with normal kidney function. Individuals following a vegetarian diet or using the drug metformin were shown to have statically depressed vitamin B12 levels, and this may increase the risk of cognitive impairment. (32) Considering that 78 million prescriptions were written in 2017 for metformin, don't be shocked if we see commercials in 20 years shouting, "Did you take the blood glucose lowering drug metformin? Were you diagnosed with cognitive impairment? You may be entitled to financial compensation." (59)

In addition to B12, animal-based food sources are incredibly dense in several other B vitamins including B1, B2, B6, niacin, and folate. (9)

Vitamin D is crucial for bone development. As people are spending more time indoors, vitamin D deficiency is becoming increasingly common. There are two forms of vitamin D, vitamin D2 and vitamin D3. Studies show that the body is best able to utilize vitamin D3. (10) Processed carbohydrates such as cereals and even fruit juices are often fortified with Vitamin D2, which is not well absorbed. Fatty fish such as mackerel and salmon as well as salmon roe and oysters are excellent sources of D3. Beef liver and eggs also contain D3.

VITAMIN D2

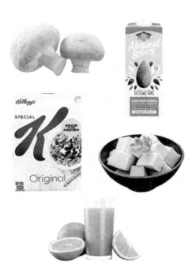

VITAMIN D3

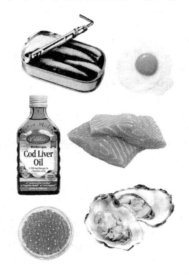

Used to fortify foods	Can be synthesized from sun
Moderately raises blood levels	Significantly raises blood levels
Levels back to baseline at two weeks	Levels peak at two weeks

Let's take a minute and talk about iron. Red meat is a dense source of heme iron. As someone who struggled with severe anemia for many years, I understand how crucial heme iron, the iron found in animals, is for the human body. How much better is heme iron, found in animal tissue and organs, absorbed than the non-heme iron found in plants? Heme iron is 2-3 times more absorbable than non heme iron. As an added bonus, while you're absorbing all that heme iron you won't have to worry about any of the antinutrient baggage such as phytates, oxalates, and lectins, attached to non-heme iron that comes with plants.

I was shocked to find out that anemia is the most common mineral deficiency in the United States and throughout the world. Anemia affects more than 25% of the world population, and almost 50% of all preschool children in the United States. Iron deficiency is no joke. It can lead to severe inflammatory disease, chronic heart failure, cancer, and inflammatory bowel disease. (11) Early signs of iron deficiency include fatigue, light headedness, and shortness of breath.

In 2011, I became so anemic from overconsumption of processed carbohydrates and underconsumption of animal protein, that I couldn't climb a flight of stairs. I fell asleep on my keyboard and woke up to a 12-page email of the letter "s" I had typed with my face while asleep. I would go on to require five iron IVs over the course of several weeks. This immediate iron boost helped me feel significantly better, but within 12 months my ferritin and iron stores were down again. I was told by my family doctor I may just "be genetically unable to store iron well." Since switching to a meat-based diet and eliminating most carbohydrates, *my iron and ferritin stores are the best they've ever been!*

I can't help but wonder if our pre-teens and teenagers who are "so tired" all the time are just low in iron stores. What about our toddlers and preschool children? Are they regularly eating burger patties, liver pate, and chicken thighs, or are they snacking on cereals, cookies, crackers, and mac and cheese? Recently, plant-based "meat" products have been advertising that they are "high in iron." When it comes to absorbable iron, in red meat it is 3-14 times more absorbable than the plant-based "meat." (12)

Research presented by Dr. Paul Mason, demonstrated that iron deficiency anemia can prevent weight loss. Why would low iron prevent an individual from losing weight? It turns out iron is an important component of energy metabolism. Without adequate available iron, our energy balance is slowed, meaning we may not be able to effectively burn fat for fuel. This can make it difficult to lose weight even if someone is following a low calorie or low-carbohydrate diet.

To demonstrate the role of iron in weight loss and energy balance, let's look at a study. Twenty-one women with severe iron deficiency anemia were followed over a six-month period in which time the anemia was corrected with iron supplementation. At the end of the study, waist circumference, body weight, and BMI significantly reduced in patients after treatment compared to their pretreatment values. Without changing their diet or exercise regimen, patients were able to reduce weight and waist circumference *simply by raising their iron status.* (56)

Let's move onto another essential mineral, calcium. Often, advocates of a plant-based diet will point out how much calcium can be found in greens like spinach and swiss chard. Unfortunately, spinach, swiss chard, and many green vegetables have compounds, such as oxalates, *that block calcium absorption.* The bioavailability of calcium from plants is very poor. Recall that if the human body cannot absorb a nutrient, it doesn't matter how much a certain food contains. Like many other aspects of plants, the fact that we cannot absorb their nutrition well provides evidence that these foods are not designed to be the *main source* of nutrition for the supercomputer that is the human body.

The calcium found in plant foods is not nearly as bioavailable as the calcium found in small bony fish like sardines or dairy products like milk or cheese. (13) To get the same amount of calcium in a single cup of milk, you'd have to consume six cups of cooked spinach. (14) Depending on your tolerance to oxalates, routinely consuming this much spinach could be a bad idea. Like anemia, bone fractures are no joke. As you learned in our chapter about sarcopenia, fractures, especially in the elderly can have devastating effects on quality of life and lead to an expedited morality. Fracture rates are 30% higher in vegans than in individuals who consume animal products. (15) I used to run with a girl who followed a vegan diet. By the age of 34 she had managed to rack up seven stress fractures. For bone health, it appears wise to consume calcium from animal sources.

How about zinc? As you've seen in our chapters on mental health and eating disorders, it is clear that the brain needs meat and saturated fat to function properly. Every single individual I have interviewed for this book or for my YouTube channel had a similar story of having symptoms of anxiety and depression, as well as overall well-being, improve after adding large amounts of meat to their diets. Zinc is an important nutrient that has been linked to brain health. One study showed that individuals who were found to be deficient in zinc had significant improvement in mood after receiving twelve weeks of zinc supplementation. (57) Zinc has been documented to be deficient in the vegan population. (16)

To conclude our discussion on bioavailability, I'd like to briefly touch on EPA and DHA. EPA (eicosapentaenoic acid) is an omega-3 PUFA (poly unsaturated fatty acid) that serves primarily anti-inflammatory and healing functions. DHA (docosahexaenoic acid) is an omega-3 fatty acid essential for brain development during pregnancy and early childhood. It is also linked to improved heart health, better vision, and reduced inflammatory response. DHA's job description is a lengthy one. Among many other functions, DHA participates in the formation of myelin, the white matter that insulates our brain circuits. It also helps maintain the integrity of the blood-brain barrier which keeps the brain safe from unwanted outside influences. For development of the brain and body, DHA is crucial. (18) There is no DHA in the plant kingdom, and most studies show that vegans consume low to zero amounts of EPA and DHA, unless they take supplements. (17)

Some vegans and vegetarians will point out that the human body can make DHA from ALA (alpha lipoic acid) which is found in flax, walnuts, and chia.

Recent studies show that the conversion rate from ALA to DHA is quite low. *At best, your body can only convert 9% of ALA-DHA; at worst, your body converts 0%.* (19) Understanding the increased likelihood of deficiencies and the lifetime impacts of undernutrition in the early stages of life, it would make sense that the Academy of Nutrition would at least recommend that children, pregnant women, and our elderly include animal products in their diet. Right?

Here is the statement from the Academy, "It is the position of the Academy of Nutrition and Dietetics that appropriately planned vegetarian, including vegan, diets are healthful, nutritionally adequate, and may provide health benefits for the prevention and treatment of certain diseases. These diets are appropriate for all stages of the life cycle, including pregnancy, lactation, infancy, childhood, adolescence, older adulthood, and for athletes." (20) Due to overwhelming evidence to the contrary, I believe it is critical that we question if it's really safe and "nutritionally adequate" to follow a diet without animal products during every stage of the life cycle.

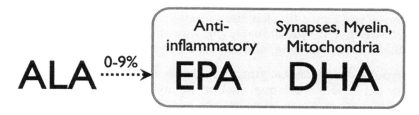

Credit: Georgia Ede

Now that we've covered bioavailability, I'd like to discuss the foods that you, and humans in general, *want to eat* consistently. This includes taste, ease of preparation, satiety, and the physical and mental health benefits of certain foods. No one is going to continue to eat in a way that causes them to be tired, hungry, angry, or depressed. If you have ever been on a diet, you have probably endured terrible tasting foods, meal replacement shakes, or "nutrition" bars. Clever marketers claim these foods contain "balanced, complete nutrition," but they are often just sugar, fiber, and some vitamins and minerals blended into a drink or smashed into a bar that tastes like chalk. Working in a hospital, I've seen dozens of well-meaning family members and friends sneak food to patients on overly restrictive, low fat, low salt diets. Humans are designed to crave certain types of foods. Our human physiology is wired to need adequate protein, saturated fat, and salt. In my opinion, it is absurd to restrict those foods and ask someone to consistently eat bland, carboard-like, processed foods or highly bitter, high fiber, gas promoting foods. Perhaps more absurd is that in the clinical setting, patients on "Heart Healthy" diets cannot order higher fat animal foods such as beef, but they can order unlimited amounts of sugar and carbohydrates.

If you have ever suffered through a highly restrictive diet, low-fat, or low-calorie diet, what happened when you lost the weight? If you're like most people I've had the privilege to interview for this book, you immediately ditched the terrible tasting foods and went back to the way you were eating before. The weight came back, and you felt like a failure! This message bears repeating: *Humans are not designed to follow a way of eating where they feel hungry and deprived over a long period of time.*

Many of the testimonies throughout this book detail heart-wrenching journeys of individuals trying to "follow the rules" of nutrition, only to experience unbearable physical and mental suffering. I'm here to tell you that if this is you too, *you are not a failure and you are certainly not the problem.* Poor nutrition advice and money hungry processed food manufactures, corporate lobbyists, and "diet" companies are the problem. It's time to use our common sense and critical thinking skills and take back our health.

For long term health success, it's ideal that the food you eat taste delicious and be satisfying. Anyone can choke down meal replacement shakes and a salad with fat-free dressing for a few months, but it's not sustainable. The first opportunity you get to sneak a few slices of pizza because "you've been so good, you deserve it," you probably will. Humans were not designed to eat in a way that leaves us longing for more food or feeling deprived.

Unless you're a professional athlete or you've recently won the lottery, you probably don't have a personal chef or the ability to designate hours every day to soak, sprout, blend, chop, or juice every morsel of food that goes into your body. In today's super busy, constant hustle society, food cannot take hours to prepare nor does it need to for optimal health. Some people have come to believe that it is "normal" to feel bloated, have stomach pain, constipation or diarrhea, or experience blood sugar crashes that cause you to crave sugary snacks. *The foods we eat are simply fuel to support our lives and ambitions.* They should not cause us to depend on them every few hours lest we have an emotional meltdown, and they certainly should not cause physical pain. You do not have to live a life where you obsess about each meal and snack. You can eat in a way that allows you to feel satiated so you can move on with your life.

There is something primal and satisfying about eating ground beef, lamb, a steak or other high-fat meats at a meal. There is a reason that you will find many people who have followed a ketogenic or low-carbohydrate, animal-based diet for years with success. Meat is ridiculously easy to prepare and leaves you full and satiated for hours. I can cook ground beef or lamb in less than seven minutes. I add salt, garlic, and I've got a nourishing meal that fuels my workout recovery and will give me sustainable energy to the rest of my workday.

Why did I always feel hungry after eating a high-carbohydrate meal, yet feel satiated after a high protein meal? I could eat up to 1,000+ calories of oatmeal, fruit, and toast and still feel the need to eat several hours later. *Research is showing that the body may continue to send signals of hunger until we consume adequate protein.* In an attempt to obtain adequate amino acids for all the important functions that protein has in the body, our hunger signals **will allow us to overeat on carbohydrates and fat** in order to obtain enough protein. Protein is that important! This is called the "protein leverage hypothesis," which proposes that humans regulate their intake of macronutrients and that protein intake is prioritized over fat and carbohydrate intake, causing excess energy ingestion when diets contain low percentages of protein. (60) This is another reason why following a high-meat diet can give you food freedom. You can easily obtain adequate protein and move on with your day. This is another reason why I don't believe in "intuitive eating" or "moderation" when it comes to carbohydrates. It's impossible to do from a human physiology stand point. *Your body will continue to send signals that you need to consume food if you don't get enough protein.* This may be why many vegans, vegetarians, and individuals on highly restrictive or carbohydrate centric diets deal with excessive hunger and anxiety throughout the day. They don't simply need more calories; they need more calories from protein.

Other Issues to Ponder

I know it's been on your mind, so let's talk about pooping. Surely, we need the fiber in vegetables to remain regular, right? If you struggle with constipation, you're not alone. Constipation, defined as a condition in which there is difficulty in emptying the bowels, usually associated with hardened feces, affects 16% of Americans and a full 33% of Americans over the age of 60. (22) I get a lot of people telling me they are terrified that they won't be able to go to the bathroom if they stop eating fruits and vegetables. While we are constantly told constipation results from lack of fiber, it actually occurs due to several facets of the Standard American Diet. The combination of highly processed carbohydrates, sugars, and lack of adequate fatty acids can cause stools to become hard and difficult to pass. Between bread, cookies, crackers, cereals, chips, pastas, and snacks such as granola bars, Americans are clogging their guts with these processed carb bombs. The main issue with fiber is it has been shown over and over again to be *ineffective* when it comes to providing bowel movements that are easy to pass, not painful, and require no use of laxatives. (23) Fiber is like an employee who for whatever reason has a reputation of being stellar, yet every time you see them, they are playing on their phone or browsing the internet. There is a false narrative going on here. In fact, one study showed that removing plant fiber significantly *improved constipation* and resolved anal bleeding. (24) I realize this runs completely opposite to everything you have heard about fiber, bowel movements, and constipation. Since adopting a high-meat, high-fat diet, I have had zero issues with constipation. In fact, for the first two weeks, while my body adjusted to the high fat content of my new way of eating, I experienced some loose stools. This resolved without any intervention, and I now have easy, consistent bowel movements. You do not need fiber to have easy, consistent bowel movements, but you do need adequate fat.

I've seen patients in the acute care setting with widespread infections from diverticulitis. Though it used to be a rare condition, diverticulitis is now one of the most common health problems in the western world. (25) Diverticulitis is an inflammation or infection in one or more small pouches in the digestive tract.

Normally, a patient is put on massive doses of antibiotics to resolve the infections caused by diverticulitis. A dietitian will be consulted to come speak with the patient and teach them how to follow a low fiber diet. This low fiber diet is high in refined carbohydrates, including mashed potatoes, white bread, white rice, and pasta. The patient is asked to follow this diet for several weeks post infection to allow their system to calm down. Then, once their system normalizes, meaning the infection is cleared and the pouches in the intestines are no longer inflamed, they are told they should include high fiber vegetables, fruits and grains into their diet once again.

Wouldn't it make more sense to eat in a way that keeps waste materials moving through the intestines efficiently, preventing stagnation and inflammation? This would most likely prevent diverticulitis in the first place. Still, the resounding advice for gastrointestinal health is to maintain a diet high in fiber from fruits, grains, and vegetables. To examine the effects of a high fiber diet on gastrointestinal health, a study of 3,950 patients looked at the relationship between fiber intake and the risk of getting diverticulitis. The study showed *zero benefit* to consuming a high fiber diet in regards to the prevention of diverticulitis. (26, 27)

Can fiber be dangerous? Recall that 25% of the world's population is anemic, and most of the western world consumes an excessive amount of grains, many of which are high in fiber. With this in mind, let's explore an article examining several studies on fiber's effect on the body's mineral stores. The article states, "The capacity of dietary fiber to bind polyvalent mineral ions (zinc, calcium, magnesium, selenium, and iron) may impart a negative effect on their bioavailability." (28) Fiber, similar to phytates, has the capacity to bind to minerals, preventing them from performing crucial functions in the body. As a population that already struggles to obtain adequate iron, calcium, and zinc, it makes sense to limit or eliminate anything that can bind to and remove minerals stores from the body.

Microbiome

Finally, we have to talk about the gut microbiome. The gut microbiome, as defined by molecular biologist, Joshua Lederberg, is the totality of microorganisms, bacteria, viruses, protozoa, and fungi, and their collective genetic material present in the gastrointestinal tract. (29) I've heard dietitians, many of whom are in love with bagels, salads, and the concept of moderation, emphatically insist that humans require the consumption of plants to ensure a healthy, diverse gut microbiome. What do the clinical trials say? Clinical trials show that *increased fiber intake does not* show increased microbial alpha diversity. (30) Similarly, studies with *low fiber ketogenic diets do not decrease alpha diversity.* (31) Many individuals following low-carbohydrate, animal-based, ketogenic, or zero carbohydrate diets have undergone fecal testing which demonstrated incredible gut alpha diversity. Fiber and plant material are clearly nonessential components to create a healthy, diverse gut microbiome.

It's unfortunate that many individuals who genuinely want to improve their health are sold probiotics or told to, "increase fruits and vegetables" in order to have a more alpha diverse "healthy" microbiome. You cannot have a healthy gastrointestinal tract while consuming refined carbohydrates, sugar, and seed oils. Adding a salad to your current standard American diet or popping a probiotic is like taking a "bad kitty" spray bottle to fight a house fire. You need to get rid of the fire and start putting in nutrient-dense foods!

Antioxidants

Well, certainly fruits and vegetables provide protection in the human body, right? Most of us have seen nuts, seeds, and berries being touted as "super foods" due to their reported ability to fight inflammation and oxidation. Wait, haven't compounds in fruits and vegetables been shown to fight free radicals and even suppress tumor growth in petri dishes and test tubes? Yes, they have. Unfortunately, as you might have guessed, the human body is neither a petri dish nor a test tube. It's a supercomputer that needs specific input to generate specific output. As humans have continued to put in the wrong foods into our supercomputers, were getting "WARNING ERROR" messages. Many people ignore these messages until the system completely gives out and we're faced with an acute or chronic illness that threatens to take our lives.

When I read Paul Saladino's book, *The Carnivore Code: Unlocking the Secrets to Optimum Health by Returning to Our Ancestral Diet*, I was surprised that there were three separate clinical studies that had been done on humans, not in petri dishes or test tubes, measuring the amount of oxidation and inflammation in their blood stream after consuming fruits and vegetables. (32) In one of the studies, participants were required to eat 10 servings of fruits and vegetables a day. That's a lot! In all three studies, the researchers thought they would be able to demonstrate that eating "nutrient-dense" plant material would show several beneficial effects in the human body. Guess what? It didn't. Investigators ran the control groups and the high fruit and vegetable eating groups through a battery of tests, and they found no difference in the inflammation, oxidative stress, and DNA damage between very high fruit and vegetable intake and very low fruit and vegetable intake. (33,34,35)

That's disheartening to everyone who has been choking down kale salads and bitter berries. To add icing to the proverbial cake, a 10-week study actually showed *marked improvements* in DNA damage and oxidative stress in the group that didn't have any fruits and vegetables. The researchers in this study concluded: "The overall effect of the 10-week period without dietary fruits and vegetables was a decrease in the oxidative damage to DNA, blood, proteins, and plasma lipids, concomitantly with marked changes in antioxidative defense." (36) Has *your* head exploded yet?

If you are suffering with any of the maladies that we have reviewed, I believe you owe it to yourself to see if ditching the carbs, at least for a set period of time, and nourishing your body with nutrient-dense animal protein can help you heal.

Since 70% of the United States population is overweight or obese, it's likely that some individuals reading this book are hoping to utilize a way of eating that results in weight loss. Can you lose weight on a vegan or vegetarian diet? Absolutely. Often people will go on vegan or vegetarian diets and initially drop highly processed, high-carbohydrate foods that are common in the Standard American Diet. Getting rid of these foods reduces carbohydrate and calorie intake and this reduction can lead to weight loss.

Hopefully your goal isn't just weight loss but fat loss. It's important to understand that high-protein diets that are either lower in carbohydrates or lower in fat lead to an increased amount of fat loss. People tend to eat until they are full, and protein is the most satisfying macronutrient because it has a direct effect on the hormones that regulate your appetite. A study looking at the immediate and long-term effects of protein concluded, "High-protein diets in both hypo- and normo-caloric conditions have shown to improve body composition, whereas in combination with hypercaloric conditions does not seem to increase fat mass, when the excess energy comes from protein."

This is fascinating! For years we've been told by well-meaning health professionals that we simply must "eat less and move more." This study demonstrates that people could literally eat the same number of calories, they just had to eat less calories from either carbohydrate or fat and more calories from protein. Even when people took in more calories than they needed, if the calories came from protein sources, they did not gain fat." (38) This provides excellent evidence that we should be consuming lots of high-quality protein from animal sources.

MORE THAN JUST
PROTEIN

BEEF
IRON
CREATINE
CLA
SELENIUM
VITAMIN B12

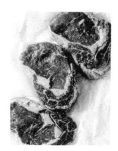

SALMON
OMEGA 3
POTASSIUM
SELENIUM
VITAMIN B6
VITAMIN D

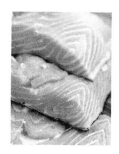

EGGS
BIOTIN
RIBOFLAVIN
FOLATE
VITAMIN B5
VITAMIN K2

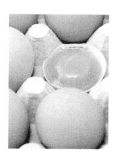

PORK
PHOSPHORUS
THIAMINE
RIBOFLAVIN
SELENIUM
VITAMIN B6

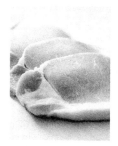

Finally, it is imperative that we discuss the effect of animal agricultures on the planet. While industrial farming degrades the soil and compromises animal welfare, many farmers are looking towards a radically traditional approaching to farming called regenerative agriculture. One thing to understand about regenerative agriculture is that it uses the natural cycles of life to raise animals with exceptional animal welfare, it has minimal waste, and as you will see in the graph below, it can sequester carbon in the soil. A regenerative farm in Bluffton, Georgia, called White Oak Pastures, utilizes every part of the cow. The animal blood is used for fertilizer. The bones are used in stocks, soups, and for dog chews. The collagen and tendons can be ground and used as compost, and the hides are used to make clothes and wallets. *It's a nose to tail practice that is actually improving the soil through its farming practices.* Look at the graphs below to see how White Oak Pastures' beef has a negative net carbon footprint.

Carbon footprint breakdown per kg of White Oak Pastures' beef

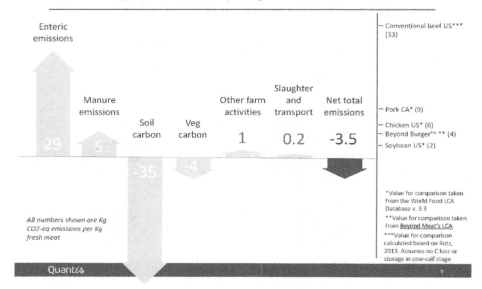

This graph shows how White Oak Pastures' beef compares to plant-based meats. Eating beef being raised through regenerative agriculture is good for the soil and good for the planet.

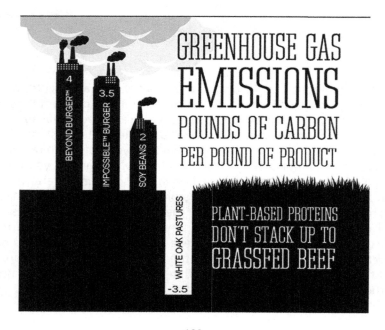

Before we elaborate on regenerative agriculture, let's get something out of the way. Plant agriculture kills billions of animals. It's been estimated that up to 7.3 billion animals are killed every year in harvesting crops. (37) While a vegan or vegetarian may not be directly eating a nutrient-dense animal product such as muscle meat from a cow, harvesting their soy (for tofu) or quinoa or kale causes the death of billions of mice, gophers, rabbits, and birds. Industrial monocropping is devastating to animal health, the soil, and the environment.

Most people are completely removed from how our food is raised, slaughtered, and processed. Many people have never hunted, fished, or butchered an animal. All life requires death. This is an inescapable fact of how the world works. We've all seen images of animals in large, multinational factory farms. The conditions are horrific, the animals are suffering, and the land will be eroded and destroyed. Every human with an ounce of compassion and empathy is against cruelty to animals and destroying the land. Contrary to what many anti-meat advocates want you to think, many farmers care deeply about the health and wellbeing of their animals.

If we want to protect the environment, it seems to make sense that we exist, which includes eating, in a way that allows the soil to regenerate, creatures to thrive, and humans to be fully functioning and healthy. Many people genuinely believe that buying avocados and bananas shipped from halfway around the world and chowing down on a vegan meat burger made in a factory in Silicon Valley is good for their bodies and the planet. Crops grown thousands of miles away and any food product produced in a lab will likely not be regenerating soil and sequestering carbon. Shipping plants around the world and creating "fake meat" products creates a relatively large carbon footprint. Industry and transportation are the two largest contributors to greenhouse gases. (41) Eating a diet that relies heavily on both transportation and industrial made foods contributes to the worst offenders of greenhouse gasses. If we truly care about the planet, we need to keep thriving ecosystems thriving, and that starts by supporting local, regenerative based farmers as much as possible.

Proper grazing of ruminant animals serves to make the soil better. When cows, sheep, and lamb can freely roam the grasslands, they improve the soil with their manure. The better the soil, the greater the carbon carrying capacity. (39, 40) The greater the carbon capacity, the healthier the soil. It's a perfect cycle. This was how nature functioned before large industrialized factory farms took over.

Big, multinational meat companies will (likely) always be able to make things cheaper and more convenient. Multinational meat companies can buy grass fed beef from any country and market it as "USDA grass fed beef," due to labeling loopholes. We cannot rely on legislation or simply take the word of companies telling us they are "doing the right thing." I believe we must take the time to research and learn about farmers utilizing regenerative agriculture. My wife and I purchase our beef from Kookoolan Farms in Yamhill, Oregon. You can see their testimony on page 187. We have spent a good amount of time at the farm, and we had an opportunity to tour the facility and speak with the owners. I hope you take the time to visit the website of White Oak Pastures to see a detailed description of their farming practices. If this interests you, go to your local farmers market and ask a local farmer if you can take a trip out to their farm on the weekend. Spending the time and money to invest in meat raised by a local farmer, or if unavailable in your area, having meat shipped from a farmer doing regenerative practices is one of the best things you to support the health of the soil and of our diminishing ecosystems. *We must actively reject misinformation demonizing all forms of animal agriculture.* Instead, we must actively seek to educate ourselves and support farmers who are practicing regenerative agriculture. Our health and the health of planet depends on it.

Finally, I'd like to address the cost of meat. I've heard people say, "Meat is **SO** expensive." This is false. When it comes to where Americans spend our money on food, it is mostly from eating out. In 2017, 53% of our food dollars went to dining out. (61) Per ounce, beef is cheaper than fancy coffee drinks, name brand chips and cookies, and even organic strawberries or blueberries. I encourage you to shift your thinking. Instead of thinking, "Meat is so expensive," ask yourself, "If eating meat truly changes everything about my health, how can I make this work? Would I be willing to potentially spend a little bit more money up front if it meant I could walk my daughter down the aisle, play with my grandkids, and enjoy a robust quality of life?" For the record, one overnight stay in the hospital runs about $11,000 which would buy a lot of ground beef. You might be surprised to find you are actually saving money by eating less produce and processed foods.

Whew, this has been quite the ride! I hope you've enjoying learning about a different approach to nutrition. I hope I've made a case that this way of eating aligns with human physiology, can be regenerative for the environment and can potentially restore physical and mental health. Now, let's talk briefly about how you can get started.

Rebekah Farmer

Instagram @tailoredketohealth
Health Coaching: https://rcfarmer18.wixsite.com/tailoredketohealth

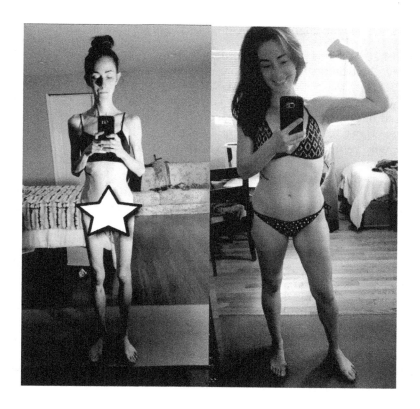

I was diagnosed with osteoporosis in sixth grade, followed by a host of mood disorders by 7th grade. I was put on Adderall, clonazepam, and Ambien and took them for 13 years until my central nervous system finally burnt out. I continued to get worse over the years, but I didn't think that not taking these medications was an option for me. It was the only option I was given!

I was diagnosed with chronic Lyme disease in 2017, when I became totally bed-bound. I had regular anxiety and suffocation attacks. I was prohibited to work due to medical instability. All of my other friends were graduating college and getting engaged. I have spent obscene amounts of money on out-of-pocket treatments and supplements. I lived in New York City for a month getting ozone therapy. I followed a ketogenic diet but still I lived in this cage of autoimmune disorders, digestive issues, and a very low level of cognition.

I started to lose rapid amounts of weight, which continued until I was at and sometimes below 70 lbs. at 5 foot 6. I was misdiagnosed with an eating disorder and actually held against my will in a hospital to be treated for an eating disorder. I came out with several more autoimmune issues and even worse than I already was. I was finally tested for C. diff and diagnosed with chronic C. diff, as I was resistant to all 13 rounds of antibiotics. I had three fecal transplants, and still was unable to inoculate this very serious infection.

In May of 2019, I was in my third emergency room back-to-back, begging for help. My electrolytes were unstable on a regular basis, and I was needing glucagon shots every day. I convinced the dietitian on staff to allow me to eat only meat. I had a very serious conversation with her about everything that I had been through and the reasons why she should give me a chance. She allowed me to be in direct communication with the chef of the hospital kitchen, who sent up multiple entrees of meat, hard-boiled eggs, and butter. I hoarded these in my hospital room as I was held in isolation and ate as much as I could. The involuntarily vomiting from ulcerative colitis stopped. No more glucagon shots needed as my blood sugar stabilized almost immediately. I gained 4 lbs. in the emergency room over the next week, until they let me go because there was simply no good reason for them to hold me any longer. I've never looked back! Within the first 2 weeks of eating only meat, my mood and energy significantly lifted. I continue to progress steadily. Healing is not linear, and there were definitely harder days, but still nothing compared to the nightmare that I had lived for the past 15 years.

I have gained 65 healthy pounds in one year. I have overcome over 10 severe autoimmune issues, confirmed with labs. Many of these diagnoses were said to be chronic. I was told that I would not live past 30 years old. Here I am today, thriving more than I ever have before. I am free, and I have been saved by faith and meat. I have learned how to have Grace with myself and I now am able to help others who are also fighting for wellness and health.

I have also learned that "Where the mind goes, the man follows." Affirmations have become a daily part of my self-care. There is true power in renewing the mind. Physiological changes manifest when we speak truth and healing out loud over our own lives. Gratitude practice changes our perspective and also creates true biochemical reactions and changes. At first, I had resistance to these things. It challenged me and taught me to dig deeper and really think about what I truly believed. It challenged my faith and was my Saving Grace.

Now, I cannot help but smile even before I open my eyes in the morning. I am so grateful to be alive and to be thriving. I am FREE!

It is such an honor to walk alongside other Warriors during their own healing journey and to be able to relate to them on a level that not many others cannot. If I had not gone through everything that I did, I wouldn't be able to fulfill God's calling on my life. I also never would have understood God's true love for me. I don't think I ever would have given carnivore a full chance if I had not come to such a place of desperation. I truly believe that we are all incredible bio-individuals and thrive in various ways. There is no one diet that fits all. Systemic healing is not a quick fix - it's a lifestyle change. And it is always worth it!

Embrace adversity, and never give up!

List of Diagnoses: Osteoporosis, cachexia, sarcopenia, failure to thrive, costochondritis, OCD, anxiety, insomnia, narcolepsy, depression, ADHD, fibromyalgia, Addison's disease, Hashimoto's hypothyroidism, central sensitization syndrome, scoliosis, chronic Lyme disease, true celiac disease, non-epileptic seizures, ulcerative colitis, CREST Scleroderma, lupus, chronic C. diff, Raynaud's syndrome, rheumatoid arthritis, peripheral neuropathy.

White Oak Pastures: Regenerative Farming

Instagram: @whiteoakpastures
Website: https://www.whiteoakpastures.com/

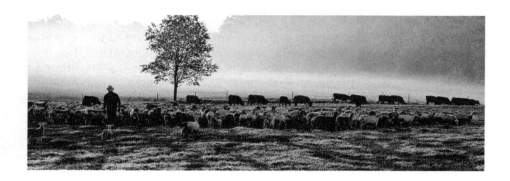

White Oaks Pastures is **Radically Traditional Farming.** Every day, we butcher meat from animals raised in a regenerative manner using humane animal management practices. This is no easy task, but it is our passion. To operate our vertically integrated, zero waste model, it takes 155+ caring people working together to accomplish a common goal: taking care of our land and livestock.

White Oak Pastures is a Zero-Waste Farm. We sell the meats and poultry we butcher on our farm to passionate consumers who care about the animals, land, and community. The hides from the cattle we slaughter are dried for pet chew rawhides or tanned and crafted into leather goods. The fat from our cattle is rendered down to create some of the purest tallow products available. Inedible viscera is composted to later be spread on our farm as rich organic matter to fertilize the soil

In soil we trust. Farming must not only be sustainable; it has to be regenerative.

Land is meant to be a living thing. It contains the natural order of all living things: Life, Growth, Death, Decay, Life, Growth, Death, Decay. The land is our teacher. Looking back to the evolution of our ecosystem informs the way we manage land today. The energy cycle, carbon cycle, mineral cycle, microbe cycle, and water cycle have all co-evolved with plants, microbes, and animals since our planet's creation. Our passion is to create an environment that allows these cycles to flow freely: microbes feed plants which feed the animals which spread urine and feces to microbes which feeds the plants which feed the animals.

Kookoolan Farms: Regenerative Farming

Website: https://www.kookoolanfarms.com/
Instagram: @KookoolanFarms

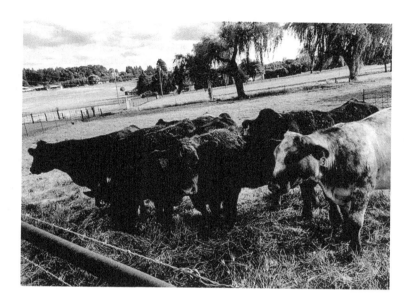

We bought this farm in October 2005; we learned to build fences, greenhouses, and barns; produced more than 80 tons of composted manure from our poultry and cattle, built raised vegetable beds; learned to raise and butcher chickens; built and licensed a poultry processing facility and a winery; bought and installed poultry processing equipment and a delivery truck with a lift elevator for driving to market; learned to drive a tractor; bought a second tractor, learned where to buy feed, alfalfa, straw, baby cows, baby chicks, the plastic bags we package our poultry in; midwifed the births of goats and cows; and have learned a lot about starting, managing and marketing a business - and about living together.

Since 2015, Kookoolan Farms is the exclusive full-time gig for both of us, with no off-farm day job distraction for either of us.

All of our practices have always been organic, but we have never been certified and have no intention of becoming certified. Our chickens eat only certified organic grains. The pastures for our chickens, beef, and lambs have never been treated with any synthetic fertilizers, pesticides, or herbicides ever. We have never used any pesticide, herbicide, fungicide or synthetic fertilizer anywhere on our farm, ever. We do not use harsh chemicals: our water is City water, and the detergents we use to clean our processing facility are environmentally friendly. Compost may be the most valuable product we (which is to say: *our animals*) produce.

Our cattle and lambs never eat any grain, only grass and clover pastures; and grass, clover, and alfalfa hays. Our electricity is 100% solar for both the business and residence. Our garbage for the entire commercial operation fits into the smallest residential garbage pickup container. All of the liquid and solid waste from our poultry processing facility is re-used right here on the farm: solids are composted, and liquids are pumped to the highest point on the property and used to irrigate and fertilize our perimeter arborvitae (legally under a permit and license from DEQ).

Our Mission:

"Our passion is to produce the best-tasting, most nutrient-dense food available anywhere, to steward our land sustainably, and to provide high quality life for the animals and people of Kookoolan Farms. We take pride in our hand-crafted foods, and pleasure in sharing our little farm with each other - and with you."

Chapter 8

Getting Started

Before getting started, I want to take a moment to validate an important point.

This is NOT easy! You are entering a battle where over 70% of the population is overweight or obese and 88% has some type of metabolic dysfunction. While the physical consequences of continuing our current eating patterns can be devastating, the dynamics of what happens on a personal level when we change our eating patterns to meet our health goals can be equally unsettling.

Sometimes, when others see people they know and love making changes, insecurity and jealousy can flare up. Curiously, this tends to happen when others are making positive, health-promoting changes. If you are choosing to go against the grain and you start to heal, this may cause others to examine the habits and patterns that aren't serving them. This is an uncomfortable process that most people would rather avoid. As the old saying goes, "Misery loves company." *Do not be discouraged if others scoff at your goals or new way of eating.* You may have well-intentioned people tell you that eating fat is bad for your heart or make witty statements like, "I'd rather die than give up cake." As you've seen throughout this book, there is a great deal of misinformation out there, and many people utilize food as a coping mechanism in times of stress or uncertainty.

I validate that it might feel difficult and anxiety provoking to visualize going through the day without certain treats, especially if these treats have become a habitual source of stress relief. I encourage you to keep in mind that this is a process not a contest. There are no winners or losers on the journey towards health. *The ultimate goal is to find what way of eating best supports your health and your goals.* While you will likely find a foundation of eating that works for you, the nuances will move and evolve as your life and goals move and evolve.

You may find that a certain way of eating works really well for you initially, and then after several months, you may want to move tiers or adjust. If something isn't working, if your goals change, or if your intuition says it's time to add or remove foods, I encourage you to be open and flexible.

Before you head to your local farmers market, regenerative farm, or grocery store, I want you to take out a piece of paper and write down *why* you are making this change. Please, do not skip this step. Be as specific as possible. In fact, I encourage you to take some time to really think about *why you want to change the way you are fueling your body.* Please note, that this is not a time for judgement. If you engaged or are engaging in emotional eating, your habits were likely serving the purpose of coping with stress or trauma. If you followed a low-fat, high-carbohydrate diet and have been dealing with GI distress, or have become overweight or diabetic, you were likely doing the very best you could with the information and resources that were available to you.

This isn't a time to blame yourself or anyone else. This is a time to take your power back. This is the time to take the first step in becoming the best, most authentic version of you. I believe this process starts with restoring your physical and emotional health through shifting the foods you eat and do not eat. Be prepared to experience a myriad of emotions when you shift how you eat. This is normal, and I think it's a really good thing. This means you care and are hopeful for a better outcome than you are currently experiencing.

When writing your *why*, it's crucial that your reason for change resonate deeply within *you*. Long term change rarely occurs if the reason for change is superficial or done for the sole purpose of pleasing or appeasing someone else. Doing something for any other reason than for what resonates deep in your heart tends to be difficult to see through, short lived, and can cause harbored resentment.

This is not to say that others don't factor into your *why*. My wife is the most important person in my life, and I am well aware that my being a physically healthy and emotionally stable person has a direct, positive impact on her and her wellbeing. What I am saying is I would caution having your *why* be something like, "So I can be a better husband/wife." Or, "So I can look good for my husband/wife." While we all want our intimate partners to be proud of us and think we're sexy, your reason for shifting how you eat may lead to a better outcome if it feels true and real to you.

Be ready for your inner critic to start speaking up! Human beings are wired for safety, and doing things outside our comfort zone is inherently unsafe. When your mind tells you that you're too old, too sick, too fat, too weak, too poor, not intelligent enough, too busy, or the million other excuses your mind will inevitably come up with, it's helpful to be focus on *your reason and commitment for doing this in the first place.*

Remember that progress is not linear, meaning that you will have difficult times and setbacks. The goal is to learn from setbacks and keep moving forward. When I first started eating a lower carb, animal-based diet, I recall asking myself, "Why will this be any different than other times I have tried to shift my eating? Am I being selfish for not just "being ok" with how my life is at the current moment?" Be ready for your inner critic and the vocal criticism of others.

Next, it is important to note that if your health is failing, it likely didn't happen overnight. In order to have continued success with anything in life, you have to follow the laws of nature. Radical change takes time and consistency.

On the road to achieving anything of value, there are no shortcuts. That is what makes embracing the grind incredibly gratifying once you reach your goals. If you've ever achieved something that you put your heart and soul into, you know it took an incredible amount of time, consistency, and sacrifice, but by God, it was worth it!

Instant gratification is just that; it's instant and it fades quickly. Like a fling with an attractive, yet dramatic and unstable person, you experience an incredible high one minute, and then the next minute you question your life choices and feel significantly worse than you did before. That is the opposite of what we are going for here. We are on a journey to take back and restore our physical and mental health. We are choosing to do this in a way that is sustainable so we can stick with it for the long haul and fall in love with the process.

If you find yourself scared or intimidated by the idea of "giving up" certain foods for a period of time, remind yourself that this is a process, and you can take it one step at a time. As we stated above, the human brain is wired for comfort and safety. If you believe you are going to be deprived or restricted, you will likely start planning your escape. Once your brain and body are consistently provided with adequate amounts of amino acids, saturated fat, and highly bioavailable vitamins and minerals, you may find a sense of peace with food that you didn't know was possible.

The "secret" to completely turning your life around isn't particularly sexy. There are no pills, potions, or 6-minute ab videos that will make you physically vibrant and emotionally grounded. The secret is simply taking the correct information, which is information that aligns with human physiology and works for your lifestyle and goals, and implementing it.

In order to be successful over the long term, I encourage you to be willing to take complete responsibility for your life. If you have suffered abuse, lost a job, lost physical or mental capacity to an illness or accident, or have had your heart broken, it's easy to take the victim mentality. Take the time to be sad, process emotions, and find support. Everything that happens to you can be used to move you towards your goal or can be used to move you away from your goal. It's all in how you frame your situation, and how you react to the circumstances (difficult and rewarding) that happens to you. *You get to choose, and that's where the power lives.*

Each person is different, and while the *general concepts of nutrition for human physiology are the same*, each person's needs can vary, depending on their current health, the foods they are able to tolerate, and their goals. As a runner, my body may effectively use more carbohydrates than someone who doesn't run. A woman or man who struggles with sugar or carbohydrate addiction may find it is best to avoid carbohydrates entirely for their lifetime. A man or woman recovering from an eating disorder may initially require an incredible number of calories (in some cases 5,000+) for months to heal the damage of years of starvation or purging. Someone may easily tolerate eating some fruits, nuts, or vegetables, while those foods activate serious autoimmune responses for another individual. You get the idea. It would be silly for me to write a meal outline that would work for everyone, because no such meal outline exists.

If you have a condition that requires medication, especially diabetics taking insulin or any blood glucose lowering drug, *you must work with your doctor to titrate off the carbohydrates and potentially reduce medications. Taking insulin or blood glucose lowering drugs without eating carbohydrates can be life threatening.* I find it incredibly encouraging that many doctors are now able to discuss reduced carbohydrate meal options with patients. Dr. Robert Cywes and Dr. Tony Hampton, both featured in this book, are two physicians leading the way in discussing the benefits of low-carbohydrate nutrition.

On the following pages, I will break down three tiers to a lower carbohydrate, animal-based eating style**. I will discuss the pros and cons of each tier.

Tier One: a carnivore, animal protein-based way of eating

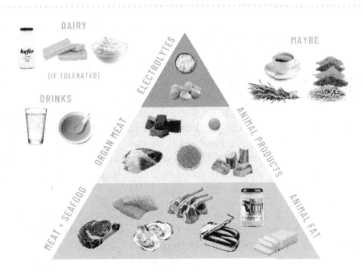

Pros: This way of eating is simple. It provides highly bioavailable nutrition including protein and saturated fat. This way of eating is excellent for someone needing to lose weight, has an autoimmune condition, or has a dysfunctional relationship with food such as struggling with sugar or carbohydrate addiction.

This way of eating can pave the way for food freedom as you are encouraged to eat until full, and you eat large, satiating portions of meat and fat.

Cons: If you are coming from a very high carbohydrate diet, switching to this way of eating may initially cause fatigue, and flu like symptoms as your body shifts from burning mostly sugar to burning fat. This can be mitigated by supplementing with electrolytes. This way of eating can cause weight loss due to the filling nature of animal fat and protein. This may not appropriate for someone who is underweight. This way of eating completely eliminates fruits and vegetables, which some people tolerate and enjoy. Spices and coffee are optional.

*Note: If you choose to start in Tier One, you may need to eat much larger portions of meat and fat than you have in the past. Most of your calories are coming from meat and fat instead of carbohydrates and sugar. Meals cannot consist of small portions such as 2-3 ounces of meat, or 1-2 eggs. I personally found it quite liberating to eat very large portions of meat and big spoonful of tallow or butter.

Sample Meal Outline:

Meal 1: 1+ pound of ground beef cooked in tallow with salt + 1-2 ounces of beef or lamb liver*

Meal 2: 6 eggs cooked in ghee (cheese optional) with butter and salt

Meal 3: 1+ pound of salmon or pork chops cooked in butter and rosemary with salt

Extras: I recommend consuming an electrolyte beverage during the transition process. There are several good keto electrolyte drinks on the market. I use LMNT Recharge electrolytes, and I've used Keto K1000 in the past.

Some people find that they only need two meals a day because they aren't as hungry. Some people find, especially after months or years of undereating, that they need more meals or larger portions. I've spoken with women who consume 3+ pounds of red meat a day for several months. You will need to find what works for you.

*Liver is cheap, and it's a nutritional powerhouse of highly absorbable vitamin A, E, K2, B9, B12, C, riboflavin, niacin, biotin, zinc, copper and manganese. (1) Unfortunately, it's quite the acquired taste. In my opinion, most liver taste pretty terrible. I do think having organ meats (1-2 ounces of liver) a few times a week is important to ensure that you are maximizing your nutrient intake. There is an excellent product on the market that I enjoy and personally use called "Beef Liver Crisps" from Carnivore Aurelius. If you find the idea of eating traditional liver makes you feel queasy, I encourage you to get online and try this product. It's a staple for me. Kidneys and hearts are other options for consuming organ meat. A recent study found that most organ meats had more trace minerals than muscle tissue. (2) Overall, liver contains the most vitamins, minerals, and trace elements between all the organ meats. With a cost of less than $3 a pound in many places, liver gives you the most bang for your buck.

DIFFERENT TYPES OF
ORGAN MEAT

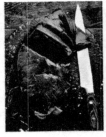 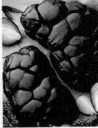 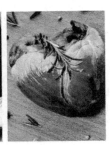

BEEF LIVER

Highest in vitamin A, E, K2, B9, B12, C, riboflavin, niacin, biotin, zinc, copper + manganese

BEEF KIDNEY

Highest in vitamin B5 + iron

Also a great source of thiamin, riboflavin + zinc

BEEF HEART

Highest in thiamin

Also a great source of niacin + zinc

Tier Two: An animal-based, carnivore-keto way of eating

KETOGENIC DIET

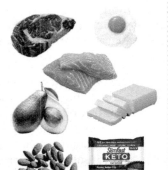

Based on limiting carbs

Plant and animal foods

Always low carb

CARNIVORE DIET

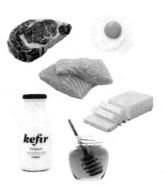

Based on type of food

Animal foods only

Usually low carb

Pros: This way of eating is simple and provides more variety than a purely meat-based way of eating. This way of eating includes nuts, low sugar fruits, and vegetables per tolerance. This way of eating provides highly bioavailable nutrition including protein and saturated fat, and it can pave the way for food freedom. If you are interested in a low-carbohydrate diet and do not have any autoimmune issues or food intolerances, this may be a good place for you to start. Many people start in Tier One for 30-60 days and then slowly move towards Tier Two to see what (if any) plant foods they can include in their diet without having any signs of intolerance.

Tier Two also opens up to the concept taught to me by my friend and foreword author, Dr. Nevada Gray. This concept is called "ditch and switch," and it uses whole foods from Tier Two to recreate traditional high carbohydrate, highly processed meals so they become low-carb, sugar-free, and high in nutrient-dense fats. In this tier, a person may be craving a specific meal, such as pizza, for example. This individual has the option to use the "ditch and switch" approach, ditching the traditional, high-carbohydrate, high-sugar, highly processed food, and recreating it with carnivore/keto ingredients. For example, a traditional pizza crust consists of mostly flour, yeast, oil, and sugar, where a "ditch and switch" crust could consist of ground pork rinds (pork skins), eggs and cheese, or ground chicken, eggs, and cheese. This tier allows you to become a creative wizard in the kitchen utilizing the foods in Tier Two. There are thousands of keto and carnivore recipes available online, as well as cookbooks. Maria Emmerich has published several excellent cookbooks that use Tier Two ingredients.

Cons: Just like with the meat-based diet in Tier One, if you are coming from a very high carbohydrate diet, switching to this way of eating may initially cause fatigue, and flu like symptoms as your body shifts from burning mostly sugar to burning fat. This can be mitigated by supplementing with electrolytes. In addition, many plant foods are problematic to individuals with autoimmune conditions or a compromised gastrointestinal lining. Unfortunately, many of us have spent decades eating highly processed foods and our GI lining is damaged. Our GI system may simply need a break from the antinutrients in plants to fully heal, and consuming plants may slow or stop the process. Starting in Tier One and moving to Tier Two may be a better option if your health is compromised.

Sample Meal Outline:

Meal 1: 6 eggs cooked in ghee w/ goat cheese, bacon, and slice avocado and salt + 1-2 ounces of liver*

Meal 2: Grilled salmon fillet with butter and salt + side of steamed carrots

Meal 3: "Ditch and switch" pizza: carnivore pizza crust, garlic butter sauce, with toppings of beef, bacon, and pepperoni

Just like with Tier One, I recommend consuming an electrolyte beverage during the transition process. See Tier One for my recommendations.

Some people find that they only need two meals a day because they aren't hungry. Some people find, especially after months or years of undereating, that they need more meals or larger portions.

*I believe in liver. See discussion under Tier One for my thoughts on organ meat.

Tier Three: Animal Based Build Out

This is the last tier. Some people may be able to easily and comfortably start here. This tier is not appropriate for anyone dealing with carbohydrate or sugar addiction. Many people come to this tier after they've moved through the first two tiers. After allowing the gut to heal and finding peace with food, some people find they need additional carbohydrates to meet their athletic or health goals. **Remember, this is not a contest.** There are no gold medals or prizes for living in Tier One, Two, or Three. The goal is to heal your body and find a way of eating that supports your health and goals.

The base of this tier remains high in fat and animal products (protein and fat), but the "build out" is very specific to an individual's goals.

While Tier One is either zero carb or very low carbohydrate, generally 20 grams or less, and the Tier Two is low-carbohydrate, closer to 25-50 grams a day, this tier allows for additional carbohydrates for specific needs. This also gives the option to supplement the diet with things like animal-based protein powder, high calorie, no sugar nutrition products, or other supplements. Please note that real, whole animal food is the base of all tiers. Any way of eating that wants you to buy mostly packaged foods or eat more shakes or powders than real food is not a recipe for long term health.

If you are in a very heavy training for an endurance or sports event, you have an incredibly active job, or you need to gain weight for health purposes or sports, it may be beneficial to take in more carbohydrates for a set period of time. This could be an excellent place to start for individuals needing to gain weight while working through the complex emotions of eating disorders.

Personally, I find myself moving between Tier 3 for my athletic training and coming back to Tier One during rest and recovery periods to allow my body a break from most carbohydrates.

The "build out" part is very individual-specific. An individual will take what foods they tolerate well and incorporate them into the plan. If you aren't sure where to start, please recall there are several health coaches, doctors, and nutrition experts referenced in this book. They can help provide guidance and accountability.

Pros: Similar to the above plans, consuming an animal-based diet provides adequate protein, saturated fat, and highly bioavailable vitamins and minerals. Additional carbohydrates can provide energy for high intensity exercise or endurance activity. Additional carbohydrates can assist with weight gain when appropriate. Additional variety can be helpful to some people. Dense nutrition bars or shakes can provide additional calories to those who are struggling with obtaining adequate calories through whole foods alone.

Cons: Grains, sugar, and refined carbohydrates may contribute to anxiety in some individuals. Additional plants (carbohydrates) provide additional antinutrients into the diet, so intolerances and/or vitamin and mineral deficiencies become more likely. For individuals dealing with sugar or carbohydrate addiction, foods containing carbohydrate or sugar can lead to bingeing.

Example of a day on Tier Three:

Becky is a 16-year-old girl attempting to recover from anorexia. She has gone through three dietitians, and has been into inpatient treatment twice. All her health care providers have recommended a very high calorie, high carbohydrate, "moderate" sugar-based diet with lots of fruits, vegetables, whole grains, and small amounts of lean protein. Becky gains weight while following this way of eating, but loses weight immediately once she leaves treatment.

She struggles with severe anxiety, diarrhea, and nausea. She recently began restricting food again and her weight has decreased. Her family is interested in having Becky implement a high-fat animal-based nutrition approach. She will be monitored by her doctor, therapist, and dietitian who values lower carbohydrate nutrition.

Becky hates the idea of eating lots of fat, but is cautiously hopeful when she hears this way of eating could potentially help alleviate some of her anxiety. She is agreeable to eat the long-fermented sourdough bread her mother makes as a source of carbohydrates. She is open to eating higher calorie foods.

Sample Meal Plan for Becky:

Meal 1: 4-6 eggs cooked in butter and tallow, 2 pieces of bacon, ½ large avocado + electrolytes

Meal 2: Open faced tuna sandwich: 100 grams of long fermented sourdough bread, spread with 2 tablespoons of butter, 6 ounces of cooked tuna, 2 tablespoons mayo, ½ avocado

Snack: high calorie supplemental food such as ½ Keto Brick or 2 scoops of whey protein in water with 1-2 tablespoons of coconut oil

Meal 3: ½ pound of chicken thighs served with melted garlic butter + 1-ounce liver pate + 1 large slice long fermented sourdough bread + 2 tablespoons of butter

Snack: high calorie supplemental food such as ½ Keto Brick or 2 scoops of whey protein in water with 1-2 tablespoons of coconut oil

In the next chapter I'll give an overview of how I train and what foods and beverages I consume in a day to fuel my running and life. You will see how I use the Tier Three: Animal Based Build Out approach.

**If you have struggled with restricting food in the past, please do not turn these suggested ways of eating into an eating disorder restriction regimen. If the thought of restriction crosses your mind, I highly recommend you invest in a health coach, doctor, carnivore or keto based dietitian, or mental health professional to keep you accountable.

I'd like to take a few minutes to go over some questions that come up when someone is pondering starting a low/lower carbohydrate way of eating.

Q: Aren't there people who function really well on a high-carbohydrate, low-fat diet?

A: Absolutely. There certainly are. Some people find they feel great eating a very high carbohydrate, very low-fat diet. For all the reasons discussed in this book, especially the fact that 88% of the American population has some kind of metabolic abnormality (that can be worsened by carbohydrate intake), I do not think this is the best approach for most people. It's interesting that many people seem to do fine on a lower fat, higher carbohydrate diet, but find they become metabolically unhealthy as they age. With the rising percentage of individuals being diagnosed with type 2 diabetes under the age of twenty, perhaps it would make more sense to start a lower carbohydrate approach in adolescence or as young adults. (3)

Q: Will I eventually be able to just trust my hunger? I'm a stress eater.

A: Many of us have spent our entire lives as war with our bodies and our intuitions. Am I *really* hungry? I think I am, but I'm not sure. I just ate two hours ago. Am I full? Should I eat again? *Can I eat again?* Am I just sad, or lonely, or bored?

We have moved so far away from a diet that aligns with what humans need to eat to thrive that we are unable to trust our bodies' signals. When you eat in a way that aligns with human physiology, you will be able to trust your body's hunger and fullness signals. This process takes some time and consistency, but it's well worth the effort. *No matter how in tune you become with your internal cues, if you struggle with emotional eating, eating foods that align with human physiology will not heal you on an emotional level.* That takes looking inside and working through your stress and trauma. This is where a mental health professional can offer valuable insight.

Q: What is the "keto flu"?

A: If you choose to follow this way of eating you will likely be reducing or eliminating most of the carbohydrates in your diet for a set period of time.

This causes a sharp decline in insulin being pumped from the pancreas into the human body. While this may be a very positive thing in the long term, this will cause the body to excrete lots of sodium in the short term. It's recommended that you consume adequate electrolytes, specifically salt, in first several weeks of your transition onto this diet. This isn't a "shake" of salt. This is several teaspoons. I believe taking a high sodium or electrolyte drink during this time can be beneficial. I highly recommend looking into brands such as LMNT Recharge Electrolytes or Keto K1000 for your electrolyte needs.

Q: Any recommendations for someone who wants to get started in Tier One but doesn't know what to buy at the grocery store?

A: As you transition to this way of eating, I recommend stocking your refrigerator and freezer with high-fat, high-meat foods that you are excited to eat. Buy the animal-based nutrition that you will look forward to preparing. My wife and I have found investing in one fourth of a cow at a time is a great way to save money. It also supports a local farmer and regenerative practices, and provides us with many delicious cuts of beef. We buy our beef from Kookoolan Farms in Yamhill, Oregon, featured on page 187. We are fortunate that each cow share includes extra animal fat, which we use to make tallow, as well as bones, which we use for bone broth and as treats for our dog, and several servings of liver. While I think it's important to eat red meat for the vitamins, minerals, carnitine, creatine, taurine, and carnosine, I absolutely validate that we all have preferences. For healing purposes, I highly recommend including red meat in the diet, but you certainly don't have to *limit yourself to just red meat.* While beef makes up about 80-90% of the meat we consume, we also enjoy pork, chicken, and seafood.

CARNIVORE DIET
SHOPPING LIST STAPLES

MEAT + SEAFOOD
Beef	Oysters
Lamb	Crab
Bison	Shrimp
Salmon	Mackerel
Chicken	Sardines
Pork	Anchovies

ANIMAL FAT
Trimmings	Duck fat
Butter	Chicken fat
Ghee	
Tallow	
Lard	
Beef suet	

ANIMAL PRODUCTS
Eggs	Bone broth
Salmon roe	Cod liver
Beef liver	Cheese
Beef kidney	
Beef heart	
Bone marrow	

ELECTROLYTES
Sodium (salt)
Calcium (dairy or egg shells)
Potassium (bone broth)
Magnesium (supplement)

Q: What if my significant other and/or family doesn't agree with the health changes I'm interested in implementing?

A: One of the greatest pieces of advice I ever received is that it's really *none of my business what anyone thinks of me as a person or what I'm doing.* Remind those around you that you're trying something for *you*, to support *your* health. Ideally, you'd appreciate their support. If they can't give you their support, that's okay too. Ultimately, you're doing this for you.

I have always believed that the best thing you can do for the people around you are to lead by example. I've had the majority of people come to me and ask what I'm doing and what changes I've incorporated in my life after they've actually seen the transformations in my overall health. Leading by example is very different than beating someone over the head with dogmatic thinking or berating them for not following something exactly as it is written. Perhaps someday someone will see the changes in you and will be inspired to make changes themselves.

Q: How can I follow a low-carb way of eating on the road or at family gatherings?

A: One huge benefit to this way of eating is the convenience of meat, fat, and plants to tolerance if they are available. No matter where you go, most places will have some type of meat or high protein item. Ten-year carnivore veteran, Kelly Williams Hogan, says she will often eat hamburger patties from McDonald's when she is traveling or having a busy day. My wife and I will often get burger patties at the airport when we travel. A ketogenic, high-meat, or low-carb diet can be easily followed 365 days a year. There are high quality, high fat, products that you can take on the go, such as the Keto Brick, created by Robert Sikes or the Carnivore Bar crated by Phillip Meece. See Robert Sikes' testimony on page 158 and Phillip Meece's testimony on page 133.

You will likely find that if you miss a meal or go additional hours without eating, you won't get "hangry" anymore. I used to be a nightmare to be around if I didn't eat every few hours. I do not believe humans were designed to function needing to snack every 2-3 hours. Cavemen didn't say, "Wait a second, Gronk, before we go on our all-day hunt, did we pack the granola bars?" When you're burning fat, you can go for hours (intermittent fasting) without eating and not feel hungry, angry, fatigued, or sad.

Q: I'm worried that I won't be able to *go*, if you know what I mean.

A: We address pooping in our chapter, Plants vs Animals, but let's revisit it here. You don't actually need fiber to poop, but you do need adequate fat. I have found that my body tolerates a good amount of rendered fat. Some people prefer to eat butter, avocado, or the fat surrounding cuts of meat. Some farms will sell suet, and many individuals who follow a high-meat diet consume raw suet. I lean towards eating rendered beef fat or butter for most of the fat I consume. I do also get fat from MCT oil, which I get from Primal Coffee Creamer, and I also get nut butter and cacao butter in Keto Bricks. Hopefully, after reading this book you will have an appreciation of how important fat and saturated fat is to the human body. If you tolerate plants well, I encourage you to enjoy them as a small part of your overall nutrition protocol. I eat iceberg lettuce occasionally, and carrots a few days a week. I do not depend on them for my bowel habits, but I enjoy them.

Q: What about vitamin C?

A: This is a serious topic and there's a lot of confusion around vitamin C. Just like LDL, context for vitamin C is *extremely important*. Many animals can actually synthesize vitamin C out of glucose, but humans cannot. We lack the enzyme L-gulonolactone oxidase (GULO) that is required in the last step of this reaction. (4) Because we do not have the enzymes required for synthesis, we must consume vitamin C. If we don't get enough vitamin C, we risk the consequences of scurvy which include fatigue, weakness, gum disease, poor wound healing, and potentially death from infections or bleeding.

How are individuals who follow a high-meat, minimal plants way of eating able to get adequate amounts of vitamin C? First, it's important to note that glucose and vitamin C look very similar from a molecular standpoint. Even more important is the fact that they use the same pathways for absorption into cells, and they compete with each other for uptake into the cells. If there is glucose present in the blood stream, glucose will win out and be absorbed over vitamin C. *In the absence of carbohydrates (glucose) far less vitamin C is needed.* If you're not eating a ton of carbohydrates, you don't have a ton of glucose circulating in the blood stream. In this case, vitamin C doesn't have to constantly compete with glucose for uptake. (4) Even though the amount of dietary vitamin C consumed on a meat-based diet is likely lower when compared to that of a plant-based diets with fruits and vegetables, *the former has a lower need for vitamin C with higher bioavailability.* Our food labeling would lead us to believe that meat doesn't contain vitamin C. It does. On the high-meat, low-carbohydrate diet, the vitamin C in animal foods plus the absence of carbs creates an environment that contains adequate vitamin C and doesn't result in scurvy.

Q: Can you follow a low-carb diet if you are a type 1 diabetic?

A: Yes, you can. I had the privilege of interviewing Elizabeth Ping (see page 49) for this book. There is an entire community of type 1 diabetics embracing a low-carbohydrate lifestyle. Many have found they are able to completely stop all fast-acting insulin and only have to use long-acting insulin. **I highly recommend working with a low-carbohydrate doctor and a health coach if you are a type 1 diabetic.** Many type 1 diabetics are finding great success with high-meat, low-carbohydrate diets.

Q: I really don't like beef. What other kinds of protein can I still eat a high-meat diet?

A: If you don't like beef, I suggest trying another ruminant animal such as venison, bison, or lamb. Some individuals who follow higher fat, lower carbohydrate diets choose to eat mostly seafood so their diet is heavy on salmon, sardines, clams, oysters, and shrimp. Eggs and cheese are other non-beef options. Pork and chicken are other high protein alternatives to beef. The food you eat should be enjoyable to you.

Q: I'm concerned about hormonal health with a low-carb diet. Can this impact female hormones?

A: Yes, eating a low-carbohydrate diet can be a nightmare for hormones *if you undereat. Do not undereat!* There isn't a lot of good data on active, healthy women and the ketogenic or carnivore diet. The only issues I've seen tend to come up when women undereat. Eat enough protein, eat a lot of fat, and *don't be afraid of adding some carbohydrates* if you find that after a set period of time, you're feeling fatigued. I would recommend against doing any intense exercise during the initial transition from a high carbohydrate to a very low carbohydrate diet. Once you have transitioned and your body is running on fat, you can add plant foods to see if your body tolerates them well. I have found that a primarily meat diet prepared with adequate fat and a few select carbohydrates supports my intense running lifestyle and allows me to have great energy, a regular menstrual cycle, and a strong libido.

Q: Can I buy all my meat at a local store? Does grass fed matter?

A: I think it would be a tragedy if an individual chose not to adopt a high-meat, low-carbohydrate way of eating purely due to the inability to afford animal-based foods that were produced using regenerative agriculture. I encourage you to buy the meat you can afford. If have the resources to support your local farmer, I think that's ideal. Check out Will Harris and White Oak Pastures on page 186 for more detail on regenerative farming.

Q: I really like vegetables. Do I need to give them up?

A: No, you might not. If your health is suffering, it may be beneficial to cut them out for a certain period of time and slowly add them back in to your diet. As we discussed in our Plants vs Animals chapter, the antinutrients in plants can cause severe symptoms in some people and zero symptoms in others. You should include the foods in your way of eating that you enjoy and that serve your health. I love my carrots and long fermented sourdough bread. I plan to continue to eat those as long as they are serving my health.

Q: My neighbor says "keto" is a fad. How can I explain to him that it's not a fad?

A: A low-carbohydrate, high-meat, very high fat diet was the diet humans followed for 3.5 million years of evolution. This is the diet that has been hypothesized to allow humans to be bipedal (walk on two feet) and to develop the large brains that we have today. (6) Many people are resistant to change or new information. I would continue to lead by example, and if/when he is interested and open to hearing you, then you can give him more information.

Q: Can I add herbs and spices to my meats?

A: If you suffer from an autoimmune disease such as rheumatoid arthritis, osteoarthritis, lupus, chronic fatigue, or fibromyalgia, I recommend you avoid adding spices for a set period of time. Do add salt! After this set time period, you can slowly add back spices to see how your system reacts to them. Many individuals without autoimmune symptoms follow a high-meat, low-carbohydrate type diet using herbs and spices without any issues.

Q: Should I fast? If so, how long?

A: Prolonged fasting of 24 hours or more is beyond the scope of this book. Intermittent fasting, where individuals eat all their meals in a 6-10-hour window seems to provide many benefits of fasting while avoiding issues that can occur during long fasts.

I believe that figuring out how to eat to fuel yourself on a day-to-day basis is likely more beneficial than completing 24+ hours of fasting (especially for pre-menopausal women). I've spoken with several health coaches who have stated that women needing to lose weight find themselves in a calorie deficit if they decide to fast too often. This can cause issues with hormones including completely losing your period. My friend, yoga instructor, and meat-based diet advocate, Sarah Kleiner, has a YouTube series where she dives into this topic. Check out her channel, "Carnivore Yogi." *If you are recovering from an eating disorder, or the idea of fasting causes emotional turmoil, or you need to gain weight, I discourage ALL fasting, including intermittent fasting.*

On the flip side, there is evidence that fasting can be a useful tool in combatting certain diseases such as certain cancers when combined with other cancer treatments. (7) It's important that each individual weigh the pros and the cons for longer periods of fasting for their specific health needs.

Q: I have tried eating more protein in the past, and my body seems to struggle with digesting meat. Is there anything I can do about this?

A: Due to years of popping antacids and proton pump inhibitors, some individuals have chronically low stomach acid. It may take a while for the body to respond to eating higher protein foods. In this case, an over-the-counter Betaine HCL supplement, taken with high protein meals, can be useful.

Q: Do you have cheat meals?

A: I truly enjoy what I'm eating. I have structured the way I eat to include foods that I enjoy and crave. Eating very processed, sugar dense foods such as a grocery store cookie or slice of cake increases my anxiety exponentially, so I rarely eat foods like that. However, you will be able to find what works for your journey and implement it in a way that allows you to feel nourished and satiated. I approach every day with the mindset of abundance. I am free to eat any foods I like. I choose to eat the foods that I have found that nourish my mind, body, and support my goals.

Danielle Hamilton, Functional Nutritional Therapy Practitioner

Instagram: @Daniellehamiltonhealth
Website and One on One Coaching: https://daniellehamiltonhealth.com/ workwithme
Podcast: Unlock the Sugar Shackles

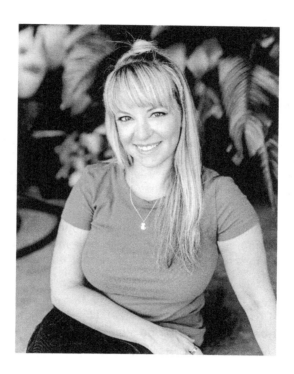

My journey began after I left my 14th visit to a doctor in a single year when I realized I was *sick and tired* of being *sick and tired*.

My diet growing up was like any other kid in the US, except I was really picky and seemed to prefer all the sweet things. My favorite foods and staples in my diet were cereal, oatmeal, granola bars, pancakes (mmm, my favorite), colorful and sugary yogurts, chocolate milk, chicken fingers, pasta, cookies, and ice cream.

I was a pretty sickly kid (eczema, strep throat, frequent colds, tons of ear infections) and always struggled with my weight. As I got older, I switched to "whole wheat" and "diet" foods but the sweet tooth was always there and my diet was very heavily carb based.

I also continued getting sicker. I had to get my tonsils out at 18 after getting Strep throat 6 times in a year (and by then had become resistant to amoxicillin). The next year I developed severe seasonal allergies and asthma. I was on 3 prescription meds and 2 inhalers. I had to get allergy shots and because I was allergic to so many things, I had to get 3 shots at a time. A year later I developed more allergies and was now getting 5 shots at a time. 5 medications plus 5 shots in the stomach every other day... no thank you!

At the same time, I was struggling with candida, recurrent infections, and chronic sinusitis. The sinus infections on top of the allergy medications made me so tired that I just couldn't take it anymore. Something had to change.

In 2012, I read Robb Wolf's book, *The Paleo Solution,* and I adopted a real food, paleo diet. I saw huge improvements with my health and literally every one of my issues went away effortlessly. I stopped the shots and got off of all of my prescriptions! I never got another sinus infection again!

I was riding high, but unfortunately, after a stressful period in my life, I started gaining weight, getting cystic acne, and I lost my period. Paleo wasn't working for me anymore and I didn't know what I was doing wrong. I realized I had Polycystic Ovarian Syndrome (PCOS). My PCOS was a hormonal imbalance that caused weight gain and weight loss resistance, cystic acne, and missed periods.

No matter how "healthy" I ate, and no matter how much I worked out, *I couldn't drop a pound* and actually seemed to be gaining. I tried to balance my hormones and increase my progesterone but nothing seemed to be working. I was crushed.

Fast forward to a few years later when I enrolled in nutrition school to become a Nutritional Therapy Practitioner (NTP). I learned that **the foundation of all hormonal imbalances is our blood sugar balance**.

"Blood sugar balance?" I thought. "But I don't have diabetes."

Okay, so I didn't have diabetes, but little did I know, my blood sugar was completely dysregulated, and I had insulin resistance which was causing my PCOS. I didn't realize that blood sugar regulation is a **spectrum** which ENDS with type 2 diabetes. I reflected on my "healthy" paleo diet which I realized was filled with fruit, starches, honey, sugary kombuchas, smoothies, and acai bowls. I made "paleo-treats," binged on dairy-free chocolate chips, and always had to finish a meal with something sweet.

The whole time I had been missing the signs that were right in front of me. I had blood sugar dysregulation & insulin resistance that were causing my PCOS. In February of 2018, I adopted a real-food, low-carb, high-fat (keto) diet and began incorporating fasting (intermittent and prolonged). I am finally able to maintain a comfortable weight and my skin is flawless. My periods are regular and my PMS & cramps pretty much vanished. *I don't even bloat before my period anymore!*

After graduating as a Functional Nutritional Therapy Practitioner (FNTP), I decided that my mission is to help individuals improve their blood sugar issues to help balance their hormones, lose weight and feel amazing. Of course, changing your macros is only one piece of the puzzle (albeit a very big piece). The other work that I do with clients in order to help them achieve their health goals is to lower inflammation, optimize digestion and hydration, replete nutrients, get adequate movement and exercise, practice stress relieving activities, reduce toxic load, and mindset work.

I always encourage my clients to stay flexible and open to changing because our needs change throughout our lives. People often get stuck and plateau when a diet that had been working for them at one point fails to help them continue to improve. Just like when I had PCOS and tried to "paleo harder," I often see people trying to "keto harder," when sometimes the answer might be to add in some more targeted carbs, for example. Stay open and flexible to change as your body and circumstances change!

Dr. Robert Cywes

Instagram: @carbaddictiondoc
YouTube: #CarbAddictionDoc
Website: https://obesityunderstood.com/
For consultations in person or on Zoom, text 561-517-0642 including via WhatsApp for international clients

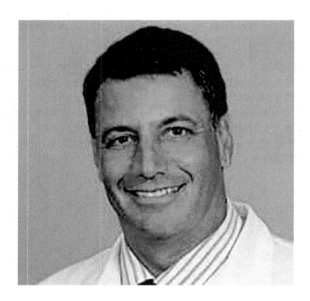

Dr. Cywes is Dual Board Certified in General Surgery and Pediatric Surgery. He specializes in Pediatric and Adult obesity, diabetes, insulin resistance and metabolic management including PCOS, Lipedema and other endocrine disorders. His focus is helping people understand and treat the true cause of their endocrine/metabolic disease including obesity and diabetes. He is increasingly working with high performance athletes as well.

Dr. Cywes received his medical degree from The University of Cape Town, South Africa in 1987. He moved to North America and studied at Ohio State University's Columbus Children's Hospital before moving to Canada where he completed his general surgery residency and specialized in minimally invasive surgery at the University of Toronto. Dr. Cywes also earned a PhD in liver metabolism and immunology and the effect of glucose metabolism on vascular endothelium injury, working with Dr. David Jenkins, the father of the Glycemic Index.

After completing his pediatric surgery fellowship at the University of Michigan's C.S. Mott Children's Hospital, Dr. Cywes was appointed as an Assistant Professor of Pediatric and Fetal Surgery at Vanderbilt University in Nashville, Tennessee where he did hepatic stem cell research. During this time, Dr. Cywes became increasingly interested in adolescent obesity and the impact of carbo-hydrates on the liver and endocrine/metabolic syndrome in young patients. Dr. Cywes' research led to a comprehensive understanding of the toxicity of chronic excessive carbohydrate consumption as the primary cause of obesity and so-called obesity-related co-morbidities, particularly diabetes and vascu-lar inflammatory disorders. In the late 1990s, Dr. Cywes understood that the prevailing treatment of obesity using a Calories In, Calories Out (CICO) model was erroneous, and he developed the Carbohydrate Insulin Model of Obesity and Diabetes (CIMOD). Using this model in combination with his understand-ing of the psychology of addiction, he developed a clinical program to treat obese adolescents using this approach.

In 2004, Dr. Cywes established Jacksonville Surgical Associates to continue his work in both adolescent and adult obesity and endocrine/metabolic treatment, and in 2013 he opened a practice in West Palm Beach, Florida. He now works with a highly experienced team of professionals from a variety of medical sub-spe-cialties to better care for obese patients. He has developed the practice into an internationally recognized Center of Excellence for obesity and metabolic man-agement. The practice uses a cognitive behavioral therapy approach address-ing carbohydrates as addictive substances to help patients manage the cause of their disease and establish remission. Based on his extensive clinical research and observations, Dr. Cywes lectures internationally regarding the physiological im-pact of carbohydrate consumption as the primary cause of the current Chronic Non-Communicable Disease (CNCDs) epidemic including PCOS and gestational diabetes. He also lectures on the behavioral aspects of carbohydrate addiction as the cause of obesity and obesity-related co-morbidities and the use of substance abuse methodology, rather than a diet and exercise approach, to the effective long-term treatment of obesity. Dr. Cywes firmly believes that metabolic disease, obesity and diabetes are not treated by surgery, however, surgery may be an in-valuable tool along the journey of becoming carbohydrate-free.

Dr. Cywes is a member of ASMBS (American Society of Metabolic and Bariatric Surgery) and is a member of the ASMBS Childhood Obesity Committee. He is also a member of APSA (American Pediatric Surgery Association). He has earned a *Centers of Excellence* designation by the Surgical Review Corporation. Dr. Cy-wes trains other doctors and surgeons to developing a CIMOD aftercare model to help patients maintain the changes to their lifestyles that they are making.

Dr Cywes has become one of the foremost authorities in the treatment and man-agement of obesity in adolescents. He recently co-authored a book, *Diabetes Un-packed*, outlining an effective approach to understanding and treating diabetes into remission. Dr. Cywes' vast experience in pediatric and general surgery serves him well in using bariatric surgery to treat obesity in adults and children.

Dr Cywes maintains an active clinical practice in Palm Beach Gardens and in Jacksonville as well as conveying the CIMOD message on social media and through his websites.

Tony Hampton, MD, ABOM, MBA, CPE

Regional Medical Director for the South Region, Chicago, IL
Website: https://doctortonyhampton.com/
Podcast: https://doctortonyhampton.libsyn.com/
YouTube: http://bit.ly/DrTonyHamptonYouTubeChannel

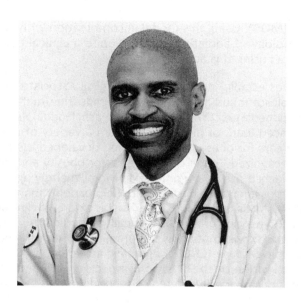

My medical career began after reciting the Hippocratic Oath, which taught me, "First, do no harm." Hippocrates also taught us to, "Let food be thy medicine." During the early years of my career, I thought that if I followed the guidance of the guidelines recommended by the experts, my patients would heal. I later learned that many of my patients, after following this advice, were not healing. Not until a family member who did not want to take medications got chronically ill, was I able to start thinking outside the box, after promising them I would help them find a way to heal. That led me on a journey that changed how I practiced medicine and how I cared for my family. I discovered that managing disease with medication or procedures never gets to the root cause of disease.

The only way to heal is to identify and resolve the root cause. So, I searched and searched, and finally discovered that the field of functional medicine was aligned with this vision. The functional medicine tree roots provided the foundation I needed to help identify why my patients were getting sick and suffering from chronic diseases. So, I decided to shift my focus to identifying the disease's root cause and using it to heal my patients. I needed an easy way to remember what those root causes were for my patients and my medical colleagues. That's when I came up with the acronyms: NEST & ROPE. I tell my patients they need a ROPE to climb up to their NEST, and both must be protected. Here's what the acronym means:

Nutrition
Exercise
Stress(less)/Sleep(more)
Trauma(avoid)/Think(positively)

Relationships(positive)
Organisms(avoid)
Pollution(avoid)
Emotions(positive)/Life Experiences (keep the ones that serve you)

I have used this approach to help patients one on one and on a broader level in my health system (Advocate Aurora in Illinois/Wisconsin).

I believe we all must work together to remove barriers to health and equip patients and the persons providing care with the education and resources they need to take charge of their health. In my previous role as medical director of the Advocate Operating System, I collaborated with clinicians and staff on programs to address social determinants of health among at-risk patient populations.

For example, I help develop education around nutrition and weight loss for the Healthy Living program that helps patients set realistic and attainable goals. The same goes for the AdvocateCare Center in Chicago (a place where patients receive multidisciplinary care in one visit), inspiring my colleagues to utilize the Center as a partner to help them manage their patients with multiple chronic diseases and improve their quality of life. I was also instrumental in the launch of the Food Farmacy (that's FARM-acy with an "F") at Advocate Trinity Hospital in Chicago to increase access to fresh, healthy food for patients and community members in need in partnership with the Chicago Food Depository. As a board-certified obesity specialist, I have incorporated that training in working with patients individually in the clinic and with small groups enrolled in the diabetes prevention program (D.P.P.). I also believe the ability to impact many patients is by leading others and serving on my organization's Governing Council, Health Outcomes Committee, and Executive Diversity Council. My current role is Regional Medical Director for the South Region in Chicago. By writing useful tools like my book, *Fix Your Diet, Fix Your Diabetes*, sharing messages on social media, a resourceful website www.doctortonyhampton.com, and podcasting (Protecting Your N.E.S.T. with Dr. Tony Hampton), I will continue to provide the knowledge to help others heal. I now use food as medicine and have become the healer I have always dreamed of being.

Temple Stewart, Registered Dietitian

Instagram: @the.ketogenic.nutritionist

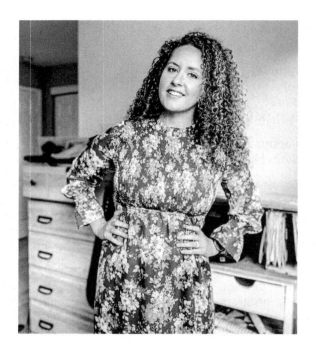

As a first-year dietetic intern at a major VA hospital, there was a lot of pressure to perform well and stay ahead in clinical rotations. Not long after I started, I began to feel very tired and experienced general soreness, acne and blemishes on my skin as well as puffiness, and noticed that my hair seemed to be falling out. As a former college athlete and a generally good eater, I hadn't experienced these symptoms before. I also realized that my workouts seemed harder; I wasn't able to lift as much or run as far or as fast. For a period of time, I just chalked it up to the pressures of the program, my recent move and general stress.

This went on for a while, but eventually became almost unbearable. As a dietitian, I wondered if my symptoms had to do with what I was eating. So, I did some research, and landed on an elimination-type diet. The first foods I took away were gluten and dairy, and I immediately began to feel better - but it still didn't solve the hormonal issues that I was dealing with.

I went to the endocrinologist; and I was diagnosed with PCOS. At the time, the only thing they offered to help treat this was birth control and metformin.

That didn't satisfy me! I knew that there had to be a food component, so I started doing a lot of research and experimenting. Two books that changed the way I looked at food early on were Jimmy Moore's *Keto Clarity*, and Jason Fung's *The Obesity Code*. When I read those books, I knew that I was going to try keto to see if it had any impact on my symptoms. The results were immediate, and had a massive impact on not only the issues I was having with inflammation, but on my underlying hormonal conditions.

After I got married, I started to experience some GI issues. At the time, I was on a semi-strict keto diet, but I had also heard of this diet called "The Carnivore Diet," that people were utilizing to heal their gut. As I dietitian, I was skeptical at first, but because I had so much success with keto, I gave it a try. The first experiment I did led me to three months of meat-only meals, and I had never felt better. Tons of energy, no GI symptoms, clear skin, and balanced hormones!

I currently eat a keto/carnivore hybrid diet, which is mostly meat-based. Without medication, I've experienced complete PCOS symptom management, and got pregnant without the use of IVF, Clomid or any other pregnancy-inducing drug. Because of my success with this lifestyle change, I now run my own business where I teach women how to balance their hormones using the ketogenic approach. I feel better than I ever have, thanks to meat!

Chapter 9

See How She Runs

When I first decided to adopt a very low carbohydrate, high meat diet, I had no intention of running at all, much less attempting ultra-endurance events. I believed that an extremely high carbohydrate diet was essential for any type of competitive endurance running. Sure, you could run *really slowly* on a very high fat, low carbohydrate diet, but I wanted to be competitive. When I adopted a high-meat, very low carbohydrate way of eating, my only goal was to reduce my searing muscle pain.

Up to that point, I believed I had done everything possible to hold onto the idea of running at an elite level. It had been a lifelong dream of mine to toe the line at the Olympic Marathon Trials race. Unfortunately, the physical and emotional suffering had become too great. I'd put myself and my wife through enough. I was physically, emotionally, and spiritually exhausted.

I didn't run a single step the first two weeks into my high-meat, low-carbohydrate diet, and surprisingly, the world didn't end. With the extra time on my hands, I did some light stretching and spent more time with my wife. During the second week of my new way of eating, I noticed my muscle pain was starting to dissipate. On day twelve, I slept through the night. At that point, I hadn't slept through the night in over two months. I could easily walk and stretch without any muscle pain. Then on day thirteen, I had one of the worst headaches of my life. In hindsight this could have been prevented or at least alleviated by taking electrolytes. Noted!

By the third week I felt happy, and I actually looked forward to going to work. I felt less bothered by difficult patient cases, and I spent extra time chatting with my coworkers. I felt calm, which was both pleasant and surprising. At the end of the third week, I began to feel an energy that I hadn't experienced in months. It was at this point my wife, who very much appreciates some solitude and reading time, told me, "You're annoying me, you should go for a run."

I was still processing the idea of not being able to run competitively. Thinking about running again made me feel sick to my stomach. If you've ever put your heart and soul into a goal and ended up deciding to change course, you can validate how difficult it can be to grieve and process the loss.

So, there I was, having the most important person in my life suggest I go for a run. The mere idea of engaging in one of my former beloved activities left me feeling terrified. What if I still can't complete a short, easy run? What if I break out in cold sweats again? What if I fail?

Then it hit me, *I could just see how it goes.* I could simply try it because moving your body feels good and getting your heart rate up is good for your heart and mood. "Drop the ego, Michelle," I told myself, "Go jog a few miles. If it doesn't go well, you can walk."

I fully intended to jog an extremely slow 10-15 minutes. I didn't know if I could jog following a zero-carb diet. I said a prayer as I headed out the door. "Well, Jesus, here we go. Let me make it 2 miles." I came back 8 miles later.

Encouraged that her spouse could run on a low-carbohydrate diet, my wife came up with the idea that we could go to a different trail every other week-end. She thought she would help me embrace my elation at being able to run again without pain. She thought I could let go of competitive running and just enjoy running for fun.

I started running short distances every other day. I was afraid that my improved sleep, muscle recovery, and overall feeling of joy might be a fluke. To my surprise, I felt great on all my runs. I ran anywhere from 4-8 miles at a relatively slow pace for me, which was between 8-8.45 minutes per mile pace. I kept my heart rate around 130-138 beats per minute.

Then, the wheels in my head started turning, and I started to dream again. I would go on runs and picture myself crossing finish lines. I could hear the announcer say, "and here she comes in a new course record... it's Michelle Hurn!" I would throw my arms up in victory and let out a primal yell as I ran by our mailbox. This earned some strange looks from my neighbors. I'm not exactly young, I turned 37 in June of 2020, but I had this feeling that I couldn't shake. I wanted to explore this renewed love for running and desire to compete.

I reached out to Zach Bitter, the current World Record holder in the 100-mile race. Check out his testimonial on page 222. I asked him if he would consider coaching me. Zach is not only an accomplished athlete, he's an incredibly intelligent and humble person. He discussed his views on nutrition and he encouraged me to take a long-term approach to ultra-running. I had been a very high carbohydrate athlete for a long time, it would take months to years for my body to perform optimally on a low-carbohydrate diet.

We also discussed how we could use carbohydrates as "rocket fuel" for my races. The goal of training with lots of protein and fat and a very low amount of carbohydrates is that my body would be able to burn fat for fuel more efficiently. This means I could burn more fat for fuel even at faster paces and higher heart rates. (1) This would allow me to spare my muscle glycogen and avoid the dreaded bonk. It would also cause less overall inflammation and oxidation in my body because I wouldn't constantly be spiking my blood glucose and insulin from eating significant amounts of carbohydrates. As I am sitting here writing this today, I am quite convinced that protein is one of the most under consumed macronutrients in endurance running. Runners are really good at hammering the gels, bagels, and bananas. In general, runners aren't grilling burger patties after runs, they are plowing through pancakes.

Zach agreed to coach me, but there was one more person I needed to check in with before it was a go.

My wife, who went from being anti low carb, high-meat to following a version of an animal-based, low-carbohydrate diet was not exactly excited about my desire to run 50 miles. "Michelle, this is the first time I've seen you *actually enjoy* running in months," she stated emphatically. As is often the case, she had a valid point. "You know I love you more than anything," she assured me. "I'm just not sure this is a good idea."

I started to doubt if it was a good idea either. Was it worth risking finally being in a good mental space? My anxiety was almost completely gone, and I wasn't in pain for the first time in years. I took the next week to journal and really examine *why* I wanted to run an ultramarathon. I discovered that I felt strangely at peace with failing. Since high school, I had put a significant amount of pressure on myself to hit certain times in races or to completely win the race outright. This time, I simply wanted to run 50 miles to see if I could do it. If I wasn't able to do it, I was okay with that too. I just had to know, if I put all my cards on the table, was it possible?

I sat down with my wife and we came to an agreement. I would start working with Zach. I wouldn't actually sign up for a race until after the Super Bowl. I'm a huge football fan, and at that time, the Super Bowl was approximately ten weeks away. If I could get through ten weeks of training, which would include running over 20 miles at a time, I'd register for a 50-mile race, and it would be a full go.

I called Zach and he officially started coaching me in November of 2019. That night, I picked out (but did not register for) a 50-mile race in Victoria, British Columbia, Canada. I marked the calendar, and I started visualizing what it would be like to run 50 miles.

Over the next 10 weeks, my wife and I took my eating, training, and living, day by day. After the first month, it was clear that I was getting stronger. Words will never do justice to the renewed joy and passion I felt during this time. It was like being a kid again. I was literally jumping over and on top of things during my runs just because I was so goddamn happy.

A major test came when I had a 22-mile run on my schedule. I met a friend out on the trails in Portland, did the run easily, and came home to help Corene with hours of yard work. In the past, hard or long training runs caused me so much physical pain that I wasn't exactly the kindest or most patient person in the hours afterwards. It's interesting how much different my mood became when I was in less pain. I'm pretty sure my wife would tell you my improved demeanor is a side effect she very much appreciates.

I do think it was helpful that I took then time to follow a mostly meat-based diet for 30 days during my initial transition to a low-carbohydrate, high-meat diet.

I did have coffee during that time. After that point, I slowly started adding in plant foods one at a time. I quickly realized certain foods caused severe stomach pain, bloating and diarrhea. I even felt achy after eating some plants, such as white potatoes. I couldn't help but wonder if some of my debilitating muscle pain and joint aches I had over the years had nothing to do with the miles I was running as a high-carbohydrate athlete, but perhaps it had everything to do with my body's negative response to particular plant foods? Maybe it was a combination of the two.

When COVID-19 hit, my May race was canceled. I was incredibly disappointed, but I regrouped, talked with Zach, and scheduled a 50-mile race for October. Then in July, the October race was canceled. Finally, I registered for a 6-hour race right outside of Las Vegas that was to take place on a 5k looped course on November 7, 2020.

The race was not canceled, and it was an honor to toe the starting line.

With 20 mph winds, but cooler temperatures, I covered 44.63 miles in the 6-hour time. That's an 8.04 mile pace for 44.63 miles. I was the first female overall and at the time I am writing this, I am ranked #2 for females in the 6-hour event in 2020. My distance covered would have ranked me #1 in 2017 and 2018. A few minutes after the race, my wife helped me find a spot to get out of the wind and change clothes. I cried like a baby, tears of joy and gratitude. It had been a long, difficult road, but I had put in the work, day after day, and I had shown myself just how strong and resilient I truly am.

Post-Race Tears of Joy:

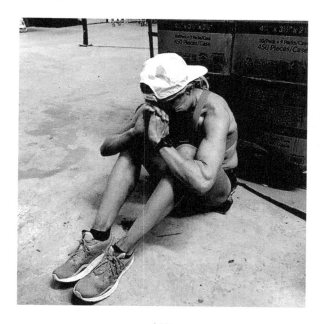

I have come to believe that eating should be something that fuels you for the things you want to do. My only two life's missions are to chase my passion and to help others. I have found that by eating this way, I'm able to pursue both these endeavors.

When I was a high-carbohydrate athlete, I averaged around 350-400 grams of carbohydrates a day. My diet consisted of a significant amount of oatmeal, peanut butter, bananas, sports recovery drinks consisting of maltodextrin and whey protein, sweet potatoes, brown rice, broccoli, chicken, salmon, gluten-free pasta, olive oil, French vanilla coffee creamer, granola bars of all kinds, and at least one large cookie daily. I ate constantly, because I was hungry constantly. I consumed three to four ounces of red meat at least twice a week.

As you can imagine, my high-carbohydrate regimen made me feel pretty fantastic for about 30 minutes after every meal as my blood sugar surged. It felt like I was getting a huge jolt of energy. The only problem was it didn't last! After about 45 minutes, insulin had caused my blood sugar to drop and I felt tired, sick, and nauseous. Eating in this way felt like I was on an emotional roller coaster. I would go from feeling euphoric to feeling hopeless. I ended up struggling with depression during this time. My anxiety increased and a visit to the dentist due to new onset of tooth pain would end in a root canal. It doesn't matter where you get carbohydrates from, they all break down to sugar, and I think it's a fair question to ask if this is the best way to fuel endurance running. Below, is an example of how I eat now during moderate to heavy endurance training. Note that during extremely heavy bouts of training, I will have an additional piece of long fermented sourdough bread during the day.

Wake up: 5:30AM (ish)

Prerun: Coffee with cream (half and half) + SFuels TRAIN drink mixed with 6 ounces of water.

Running up to 2 hours: I use water and electrolytes during the run. I will not take in calories unless we are practicing for race specific nutrition towards the end of a training cycle.

Running over 2 hours or very difficult, high intensity run: About 45 minutes into the run, I will use SFuels RACE. I mix it with 4-6 ounces of water. I will take in one packet of RACE every hour after the first dose.

Post run: Water and electrolytes. I really like LMNT's Raspberry Salt electrolyte drink.

TIP**Get your heart rate down after you work out. This has nothing to do with nutrition, but I see so many athletes go straight from a run to dashing to a shower, then dashing to work. This is a good way to spike your cortisol and keep stress hormones high. Take a few minutes to do something post run/workout to get your heart rate down. I like to stretch, do some deep breathing, and pet my dog.

Meal 1:

- ¾-1 full pound of grass-fed beef cooked in tallow + butter + Redmond's Sea Salt
- Coffee with butter, heavy cream, or Primal Coffee Creamer
- 1-2 ounces of liver or ½ bag of Liver Crisps by Carnivore Aurelius (I eat liver 2-3 times a week)

Meal 2:

- ½ pound of ground beef with butter or 8 ounces of tuna with mayo or 2 links of pork sausage

Meal two is a bit more flexible. I often eat whatever high protein item we have left over or available. I was really fortunate to work for Scratch Meats in Portland, Oregon this fall so I obtained fresh caught salmon and sausage from them.

Meal 3:

- Large ribeye steak, ground lamb, or more ground beef cooked with butter + Redmond's Sea Salt
- Carrots cooked in ghee
- Slice of long fermented sourdough, baked by my wife, with butter

Still hungry?

No: That's it.

Yes: Keto Brick or whipped heavy cream (heavy cream + vanilla extract + sea salt in a blender).

This way of eating is *very different* than what many endurance meal plans advocate. There's significantly less carbohydrates, and significantly more protein and fat. I believe it's essential to consume adequate fat when eating a low-carbohydrate diet. I prefer to eat very high-fat meats. I will add tallow to beef while I'm cooking, or I'll add butter to fish or chicken. I'll put butter on steak or burger patties. I'll occasionally use mayonnaise, and I enjoy Keto Bricks or Carnivore Bars when I'm on the go or need more calories. I eat Swiss cheese occasionally, but it's not a regular part of my diet. I'm in love with Primal Coffee Creamer. I like the idea of getting a dose of collagen protein with high quality fats every day.

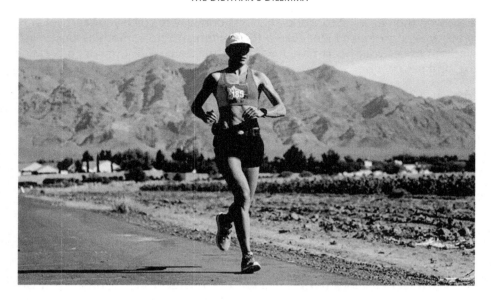

Do I deviate from this plan? Yes, sometimes I do. This is what I follow 90-95% of the time. When you find something that works for you, I highly suggest you do the same. I found it beneficial to structure my nutrition to be in direct alignment with *my goals.* I will certainly consume a lot more carbohydrates than the above plan on my race day. My only goal on race day is to run as fast as possible for as long as possible. My goal on race day is different, so my nutrition will be different.

When I first starting using the sports nutrition products by SFuels, they asked me if I would be interested in being an ambassador for them. I told them I wanted to make sure that I liked the products, they worked well for me, and I felt like I could speak authentically about them, before I committed to representing them.

The SFuels products have exceeded my expectations. I felt strong and consistent during my ultra-training and racing. I never had any stomach or gastrointestinal distress, and I've recovered quickly from one training run to the next. The SFuels products align with my purpose of keeping insulin low and allowing my body to use fat for fuel during running. I used SFuels during my first Ultra Race, and I'm excited to continue to use them for my upcoming events.

Benefits of SFuels

Our body can only store a very limited amount of carbohydrates. If we teach our bodies to burn fat for fuel, through our training and nutrition, we can avoid the dreaded bonk and improve endurance performance and speed up muscle recovery.

Following a low-carbohydrate, high-fat diet and incorporating SFuels into your training can assist the body in stable, flexible fuel burning (able to use both carbohydrate and fat versus just carbohydrate) for hard working muscles. (2-8)

Evidence suggests that a higher carbohydrate intake during training and racing can contribute to GI distress including nausea, vomiting, diarrhea (not good). When fat oxidation is increased, you need less total carbohydrate to fuel your activity. This can mean less GI distress and better training and racing sessions (very good). (2-8)

Fat oxidation is thought to cause less overall inflammation than carbohydrate oxidation. Less inflammation supports more consistent racing and training blocks. (2-8)

If you want to transition from high sugar, blood sugar-spiking sports nutrition products or you're simply looking to improve performance and recovery all while avoiding GI distress, I highly recommend you give SFuels products a try.

What if you are not an endurance athlete but are simply looking for a product to help optimize your low-carbohydrate lifestyle? Currently, SFuels has the SFuels LIFE product which is designed to be added to meals, snacks and drinks. SFuels is continuing to develop an expanded portfolio of products to support all day everyday fat oxidation.

Check out their website: https://www.sfuelsgolonger.com/

Get 5% off your first order with the discount code: MICHELLE5

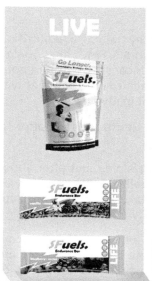
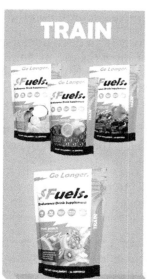
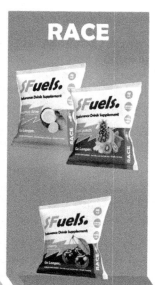

Zach Bitter

Professional Endurance Athlete & Coach
Current World Record Holder in the 100-mile Race
Instagram: @ZachBitter
Website: https://zachbitter.com/

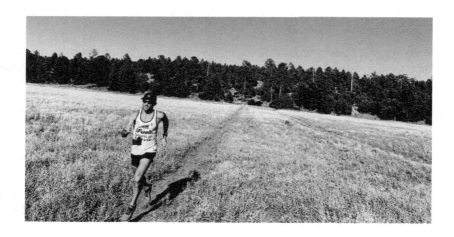

I began endurance sport at an early age. By high school it became my primary sport. I was fortunate to be able to compete at the collegiate level and continue building my knowledge base around endurance training methodology. After college, I became interested in ultramarathons.

Early on, I realized that the way I had been pursuing my training and nutrition for ultramarathons was not ideal for me as an individual. My sleep quality began to suffer, and my energy levels were wildly inconsistent throughout the day. In 2011, I decided to take a different approach to nutrition that was centered around fat being the primary macronutrient in my diet.

My sleep quality was one of the first things to return. Shortly after, I noticed a much more stable energy levels throughout the day.

It took me a bit longer to notice the changes in my training, but after about four weeks my runs at low intensity began to normalize. From there, I was able to tease out what ranges of carbohydrate intake could help execute some of the bigger training sessions and high intensity efforts.

I found my sweet spot about 1.5-2 years into the journey, when I discovered very low classic ketogenic levels of carbohydrate worked great for me on off season and recovery blocks, while reintroducing small amounts of carbohydrate around key sessions and big volume builds gave me the best of both worlds.

Since my energy expenditure can be quite polarizing depending on whether I am in training versus off season, I have found that always keeping fat as my main macronutrient works well, but not being afraid to flex my carbohydrate intake up to approximately 20 percent of my intake when my training load is highest.

Kristin Barishian

Instagram: @keto.marathoner

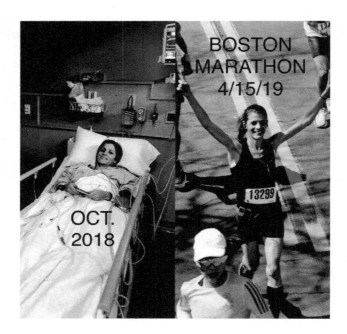

I followed the traditional low-fat diet, eating up to 10 times a day to fuel my marathon training. I would eat a full bag of rice cakes, protein powder, up to five pounds of vegetables a day, and low-fat chicken or turkey.

This way of eating landed me in the hospital in 2018. I had anemia, edema, fatty liver, and scarring on one of my kidneys. Once I got out of the hospital, I decided I had to make a change. I started the ketogenic diet. I was really afraid of fat, so this way of eating was difficult for me. The ketogenic diet is up to 80% fat, but eating this way got easier over time. I followed a strict ketogenic from November of 2018 to April 2019. At the Boston Marathon in 2019, I ran a full 15 minutes faster than my previous best marathon time. (See photo)

As much as I liked the ketogenic way of eating, I still occasionally felt bloated. I also struggled with carbohydrate and sugar cravings. I decided to make the switch to a higher meat diet in November of 2019. This is when I adopted the carnivore diet. Since following the carnivore diet, I feel like I have more energy, less anxiety, and reduced cravings. With two large meals a day, I feel satisfied. I don't think of this as a diet, I think of this as a way of life. I'm grateful for my health and this way of eating.

Dr. Nevada Gray PharmD, R.N.

Instagram: @thepaleopharmacist
Facebook: The PALEO Pharmacist
Twitter: @DrNevadaGray
Website/Blog: www.thepaleopharmacist.com

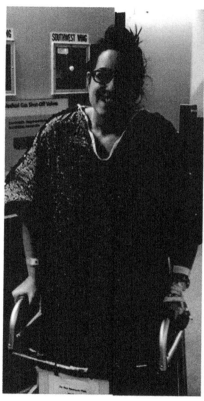 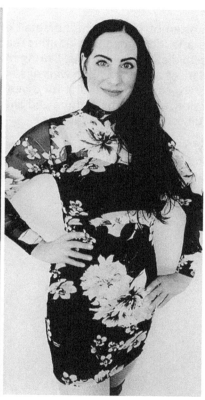

My whole life I struggled with asthma, eczema and allergies. Certain foods would make me wheeze, give me an upset stomach, or swell my lips, tongue, and throat. Unfortunately, most of these foods happened to be fruits and vegetables.

It was not until later adulthood that I was diagnosed with Oral Allergy Syndrome and gluten allergy. Due to my allergy issue, I naturally gravitated to a highly processed diet, which led to obesity and polycystic ovarian syndrome. In my 20's and early 30's, I earned degrees in biochemistry, nursing and pharmacy in an effort to improve my own health and help others along the way. Upon graduating pharmacy school, I reached my heaviest weight at 220 plus lbs. I am only 5'4".

It was at this time that I hired a personal trainer and discovered the paleo diet and embraced the eat less, move more philosophy. Needless to say, there was little return on my investment spending 2 hours every day at the gym and eating 6 small meals a day. In 2016, I herniated a disc in my lumbar spine that required emergency neurosurgery for cauda equina syndrome.

In an attempt to save the horsetail of my spinal cord, I started a medically therapeutic ketogenic diet after reading about the potential neuromotor/protective effects of ketosis. During my 2-year recovery of correcting muscle imbalances and learning to walk again, I evolved my nutrition to a protein-priority zero-carbohydrate diet for 3 years. After losing 92 lbs., putting PCOS in remission, and taming asthma and allergies, I worked with an allergist to successfully add foods back in.

Today, 5 years after my injury, I have been able to maintain my weight loss and healing with the 4 Pillars I used during my recovery 1. Ketogenic Nutrition 2. Restorative Sleep 3. A Quantum Mindset 4. Functional Fitness.

Primal Coffee Company

Website: https://primalcoffeecompany.com/
Instagram: @primalcoffeecompany
Facebook: ThePrimalCoffeeCompany

Save 15% on your order of Primal Coffee with the code: RUNEATMEATREPEAT

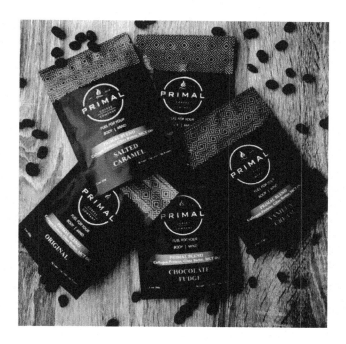

Our company was not created based on a business plan or with the intent to be profitable. We focused on ingredients we found to be the healthiest for us and created our "Primal Blend" so that we could quickly make our morning coffee without having to weigh every ingredient individually, and never run out of ingredients. However, our blend has not always been what it is today. Over time, it has evolved into what we believe is the perfect creamer for your coffee, both in taste and nutrition.

It actually all began with collagen. I dislocated my shoulder in high school playing football with some friends. Years later, my shoulder would re-dislocate again from things like diving into a pool, playing sports, or while sleeping in the middle of the night. I found my options for healing to be very limited, and I was told I would need surgery or I would just have to live with it. Upon doing some research I found consuming collagen on a regular basis could be beneficial, because as we age, injuries take longer to heal (if at all) as our bodies produce less collagen naturally. Figuring I had nothing to lose, I began to add it to my coffee every morning. Within a few months my shoulder felt stronger and no longer held constant tension. My shoulder has not dislocated once since adding collagen to my daily routine!

Everything changed when we (my business partner Cody and I) switched to a high-fat, low-carb diet with moderate to high amounts of protein. We no longer felt tired throughout the day and both felt an overall sense of mental clarity. At the time, I was still only putting collagen in my coffee, but I realized there were other products I could add in for extra fats (MCT oil powder or other variants), and I remembered how great I felt the day I tried a bulletproof coffee. Some of the products tasted great, but upon further inspection they lacked ingredients that I was looking for, or they had lots of additives, preservatives, and hidden sugars.

Cody and I wanted a morning cup of coffee that we not only looked forward to, but our bodies would as well. That's when our "Primal Blend" was born. At first, we weighed out each ingredient individually. This was very time consuming due to the fact that we were adding 10 different ingredients to our coffee every morning. Unfortunately, we would often run out of ingredients, so we decided to mix all of our ingredients together and create a large batch of coffee creamer, enough to last us a couple of weeks. After some trial and error, we were able to perfect our ratio of ingredients to create the perfect all in one powdered coffee creamer. We drank a cup (or two) every morning and due to increased interest from friends and family, we began preparing small batches to give away.

That's how Primal Coffee Company started, we both love drinking our Primal Blend in the morning and look forward to it every day, and we know others will too. We searched for the highest quality, healthiest coffee creamer, but could not find one that was good for us, so we created our own. Many hours were spent sourcing premium, expensive ingredients. Unsure if we even had a viable company, we figured worst case scenario would be we'd have a ton of creamer to enjoy for a while.

This has been a long, amazing journey. The opportunity to create what we love, and share it with others has truly been a wonderful experience! We look forward to growing and continuing Primal Coffee Company.

Final Thoughts

We began this book by asking: *What would you do if your health was restored by doing the opposite of everything you were taught?*

One of my favorite songs is *Hold us Together* by Matt Maher. It has a lyric that goes, "This is the first day of the rest of your life." Today, is indeed, the first day of the rest of your life. You get to make an important choice. Do you want to continue your same patterns, or does it make sense to make a change? Restoring your physical and mental health and beginning to pave the way to a beautiful future is within your reach. It requires the bravery and fortitude to go against the grain and the courage to be consistent.

I believe we will see a low-carbohydrate diet become more mainstream as the evidence for its efficacy continues to grow, but *you don't need to wait to get started.* A low-carbohydrate, high-fat diet is sustainable, boasts high compliance rates, and it can lead to improved metabolic health. People enjoy eating this way because the food tastes great, they aren't hungry, and they, often for the first time in years, feel *really good.*

A little over a year ago, I couldn't run more than a few miles without feeling sick and experiencing piercing muscle pain. I suffered severe anxiety, and bouts of depression. I obsessed about food constantly, and felt exhausted, achy, and bloated repeatedly after eating.

While working on this book, on November 7, 2020, I ran 44.63 miles, and I can't wait for my next race. My emotions are significantly more stable, and I feel calm and peaceful.

As I've said publicly on podcasts and on other mediums, I have no stock in what anyone chooses to eat. If people decide to follow very high carbohydrate diets, that's fine. If people feel great on vegan or vegetarian diets, I'm happy for them.

After completely transforming my health with a low-carbohydrate, high-meat, high-fat diet, and witnessing the profound disconnect between feeding people high-carbohydrate diets and watching them suffer preventable, chronic illnesses in our health care system, I could no longer be silent.

I knew I had to discuss the potentially lifesaving benefits of following a diet that aligns with human physiology. In writing *The Dietitian's Dilemma*, it was my ultimate goal to provide clear, factual information, and give each person reading it hope. Change is possible, joy is possible, peace with food is possible. I'm living proof of this, and you can be too.

Works Cited

Chapter 1: Diabetes

1. Feinman RD, Pogozelski WK, Astrup A, et al. Dietary carbohydrate restriction as the first approach in diabetes management: critical review and evidence base [published correction appears in Nutrition. 2019 Jun;62:213]. *Nutrition*. 2015;31(1):1-13. doi:10.1016/j.nut.2014.06.011
2. "What Is Diabetes?" *Centers for Disease Control and Prevention*, Centers for Disease Control and Prevention, 11 June 2020, www.cdc.gov/diabetes/basics/diabetes.html.
3. Caceres, Vanessa, and Michael Schroeder. "What's Driving the Rise in Type 2 Diabetes in Kids?" *U.S. News & World Report*, U.S. News & World Report, 9 Apr. 2019, health.usnews.com/health-care/patient-advice/articles/2017-07-25/why-type-2-diabetes-is-on-the-rise-in-children-and-teens.
4. Beyaz S, Güler ÜÖ, Bağır GŞ. Factors affecting lifespan following below-knee amputation in diabetic patients. *Acta Orthop Traumatol Turc*. 2017;51(5):393-397. doi:10.1016/j.aott.2017.07.001
5. Ellis, Esther. "How an RDN Can Help with Diabetes." *EatRight*, 13 Nov. 2019, www.eatright.org/health/diseases-and-conditions/diabetes/how-an-rdn-can-help-with-diabetes.
6. "Chapter 1 Old Man River." *Strong Medicine*, by Blake F. Donaldson, Cassell, 1963, pp. 8–8.
7. Morrison, Katharine. "Low Carbohydrate Diets for Diabetes Control." *British Journal of General Practice*, British Journal of General Practice, 1 Nov. 2005, bjgp.org/content/55/520/884.1.
8. Caffrey, Mary. "Diabetic Amputations May Be Rising in the United States." *AJMC*, 13 Dec. 2018, www.ajmc.com/view/diabetic-amputations-may-be-rising-in-the-united-states.
9. Jellinger, Paul S. "Metabolic Consequences of Hyperglycemia and Insulin Resistance." *Clinical Cornerstone*, Excerpta Medica, 23 Dec. 2007, www.sciencedirect.com/science/article/abs/pii/S1098359707800196?via=ihub.
10. U. S. National Commission on Diabetes. *Report of the National Commission on Diabetes to the Congress of the United States*. National Institutes of Health, 2017.
11. Tabish SA. Is Diabetes Becoming the Biggest Epidemic of the Twenty-first Century?. *Int J Health Sci (Qassim)*. 2007;1(2):V-VIII.

12. eatright.org. "Meet Our Sponsors." *Eatrightpro.org*, 2020, www.eatrightpro.org/about-us/advertising-and-sponsorship/meet-our-sponsors.

13. Letter, The Pharma. "According to Market Research, the Worldwide Pharmaceutical Market Was Worth Nearly $1.3 Trillion in 2019..." *TPL*, 3 Mar. 2020, www.thepharmaletter.com/article/annual-revenue-of-top-10-big-pharma-companies.

14. Schulte EM, Avena NM, Gearhardt AN. Which foods may be addictive? The roles of processing, fat content, and glycemic load. *PLoS One*. 2015;10(2):e0117959. Published 2015 Feb 18. doi:10.1371/journal.pone.0117959.

15. Volek JS, Fernandez ML, Feinman RD, Phinney SD. Dietary carbohydrate restriction induces a unique metabolic state positively affecting atherogenic dyslipidemia, fatty acid partitioning, and metabolic syndrome. *Prog Lipid Res*. 2008;47(5):307-318. doi:10.1016/j.plipres.2008.02.003.

16. Loria P, Lonardo A, Anania F. Liver and diabetes. A vicious circle. *Hepatol Res*. 2013;43(1):51-64. doi:10.1111/j.1872-034X.2012.01031.x.

17. Boden G, Sargrad K, Homko C, Mozzoli M, Stein TP. Effect of a low-carbohydrate diet on appetite, blood glucose levels, and insulin resistance in obese patients with type 2 diabetes. *Ann Intern Med*. 2005;142(6):403-411. doi:10.7326/0003-4819-142-6-200503150-00006.

18. Cunha, John P. "Side Effects of Humalog (Insulin Lispro (Human Analog)), Warnings, Uses." *RxList*, RxList, 17 June 2020, www.rxlist.com/humalog-side-effects-drug-center.htm.

19. Fontana L, Eagon JC, Trujillo ME, Scherer PE, Klein S. Visceral fat adipokine secretion is associated with systemic inflammation in obese humans. *Diabetes*. 2007;56(4):1010-1013. doi:10.2337/db06-1656.

20. Nazzal Z, Khatib B, Al-Quqa B, Abu-Taha L, Jaradat A. The prevalence and risk factors of urinary incontinence amongst Palestinian women with type 2 diabetes mellitus: A cross-sectional study. *Arab J Urol*. 2019;18(1):34-40. Published 2019 Dec 9. doi:10.1080/2090598X.2019.1699340.

21. Matthew J Callaghan, Daniel J. Ceradini, and Geoffrey C. Gurtner. Hyperglycemia-Induced Reactive Oxygen Species and Impaired Endothelial Progenitor Cell Function. Antioxidants & Redox Signaling, Nov 2005. 1476-1428.

22. Landau, B R, et al. "Contributions of Gluconeogenesis to Glucose Production in the Fasted State." *The Journal of Clinical Investigation*, American Society for Clinical Investigation, 15 July 1996, www.jci.org/articles/view/118803.

23. Ancel Keys, Alessandro Mienotti, Mariti J. Karvonen, Christ Aravanis, Henry Blackburn, Ratko Buzina, B. S. Djordjevic, A. S. Dontas, Flaminio Fidanza, Margaret H. Keys, Daan Kromhout, Srecko Nedeljkovic, Sven Punsar, Fulvia Seccareccia, Hironori Toshima, The Diet And 15-Year Death Rate In The Seven Countries Study, *American Journal of Epidemiology*, Volume 124, Issue 6, December 1986, Pages 903 915, https://doi.org/10.1093/oxfordjournals.aje.a114480

24. Miller, Anna Medaris. "Feeding Your Baby's Brain." *U.S. News & World Report*, U.S. News & World Report, 5 Jan. 2016, health.usnews.com/health-news/health-wellness/articles/2016-01-05/feeding-your-babys-brain.

25. Tasevska N, Park Y, Jiao L, Hollenbeck A, Subar AF, Potischman N. Sugars and risk of mortality in the NIH-AARP Diet and Health Study. *Am J Clin Nutr*. 2014;99(5):1077-1088. doi:10.3945/ajcn.113.069369.

26. *Tolstoi, Edward (June 20, 1929). "THE EFFECT OF AN EXCLUSIVE MEAT DIET LASTING ONE YEAR ON THE CARBOHYDRATE TOLERANCE OF TWO NORMAL MEN" (PDF). J. Biol. Chem. (83): 747–752. Retrieved 2015-12-16.*

27. Vilhjalmur, Stefansson. *The Fat of the Land*. 1956.

28. Bolla AM, Caretto A, Laurenzi A, Scavini M, Piemonti L. Low-Carb and Ketogenic Diets in Type 1 and Type 2 Diabetes. *Nutrients*. 2019;11(5):962. Published 2019 Apr 26. doi:10.3390/nu11050962.

29. Bolla AM, Caretto A, Laurenzi A, Scavini M, Piemonti L. Low-Carb and Ketogenic Diets in Type 1 and Type 2 Diabetes. *Nutrients*. 2019;11(5):962. Published 2019 Apr 26. doi:10.3390/nu11050962.

30. Westman EC, Vernon MC. Has carbohydrate-restriction been forgotten as a treatment for diabetes mellitus? A perspective on the ACCORD study design. *Nutr Metab (Lond)*. 2008;5:10. Published 2008 Apr 9. doi:10.1186/1743-7075-5-10.

31. Donald Wiebe, The Cholesterol Wars: The Skeptics vs. the Preponderance of Evidence. Daniel Steinberg. San Diego, CA, Academic Press-Elsevier, 2007, ISBN: 978-0-12-373979-7., *Clinical Chemistry*, Volume 55, Issue 7, 1 July 2009, Pages 1441–1442, https://doi.org/10.1373/clinchem.2009.128355.

32. Clarke R, Frost C, Collins R, Appleby P, Peto R. Dietary lipids and blood cholesterol: quantitative meta-analysis of metabolic ward studies. *BMJ.* 1997;314(7074):112-117. doi:10.1136/bmj.314.7074.112.

33. Orchard TJ, Forrest KY, Ellis D, Becker DJ. Cumulative glycemic exposure and microvascular complications in insulin-dependent diabetes mellitus. The glycemic threshold revisited. *Arch Intern Med.* 1997;157(16):1851-1856.

Chapter 2: Mental Illness

1. Al-Adawi S, Dorvlo AS, Al-Ismaily SS, et al. Perception of and attitude towards mental illness in Oman. *Int J Soc Psychiatry.* 2002;48(4):305-317. doi:10.1177/002076402128783334.

2. Palmer, Chris. *Human Performance Outliers Interviews Dr. Palmer - The Connection between Mental and Metabolic Disorders.* 26 Jan. 2020, www.chrispalmermd.com/human-performance-outliers-gut-microbiome/.

3. "CDC - NCHS - National Center for Health Statistics." *Centers for Disease Control and Prevention*, Centers for Disease Control and Prevention, 7 Aug. 2020, www.cdc.gov/nchs/index.htm

4. Friedrich, M. Depression Is the Leading Cause of Disability Around the World. *JAMA.* 2017;317(15):1517. doi:10.1001/jama.2017.3826.

5. Spiegel, Alix. "Children Labeled 'Bipolar' May Get A New Diagnosis." *NPR*, NPR, 10 Feb. 2010, www.npr.org/templates/story/story.php?storyId=123544191.

6. McIntosh, John L. *U.S.A. SUICIDE: 2008 OFFICIAL FINAL DATA.* 4 Oct. 2011, health.maryland.gov/suicideprevention/Documents/National%20Data%202008.pdf.

7. De Hert M, Detraux J, Vancampfort D. The intriguing relationship between coronary heart disease and mental disorders. *Dialogues Clin Neurosci.* 2018;20(1):31-40.

8. Newcomber, John. "Metabolic Syndrome and Mental Illness." *AJMC*, 1 Nov. 2007, www.ajmc.com/view/nov07-2657ps170-s177.

9. Laura E. Jones & Caroline P. Carney (2006) Increased Risk for Metabolic Syndrome in Persons Seeking Care for Mental Disorders, Annals of Clinical Psychiatry, 18:3, 149-155, DOI: 10.3109/10401230600801085.

10. Zuccoli GS, Saia-Cereda VM, Nascimento JM, Martins-de-Souza D. The Energy Metabolism Dysfunction in Psychiatric Disorders

Postmortem Brains: Focus on Proteomic Evidence. *Front Neurosci.* 2017;11:493. Published 2017 Sep 7. doi:10.3389/fnins.2017.00493.

11. Impaired mitochondrial function in psychiatric disorders. *Manji H, Kato T, Di Prospero NA, Ness S, Beal MF, Krams M, Chen G Nat Rev Neurosci. 2012 Apr 18; 13(5):293-307.*

12. Cerebral phosphate metabolism in first-degree relatives of patients with schizophrenia. *Klemm S, Rzanny R, Riehemann S, Volz HP, Schmidt B, Gerhard UJ, Filz C, Schönberg A, Mentzel HJ, Kaiser WA, Blanz B Am J Psychiatry. 2001 Jun; 158(6):958-60.*

13. The role of mitochondrial dysfunction in bipolar disorder. *Kato T Drug News Perspect. 2006 Dec; 19(10):597-602.*

14. Lyra E Silva NM, Lam MP, Soares CN, Munoz DP, Milev R, De Felice FG. Insulin Resistance as a Shared Pathogenic Mechanism Between Depression and Type 2 Diabetes. *Front Psychiatry.* 2019;10:57. Published 2019 Feb 14. doi:10.3389/fpsyt.2019.00057.

15. Hajek T, Calkin C, Blagdon R, Slaney C, Uher R, Alda M. Insulin resistance, diabetes mellitus, and brain structure in bipolar disorders. *Neuropsychopharmacology.* 2014;39(12):2910-2918. doi:10.1038/npp.2014.148.Soontornniyomkij V, Lee EE, Jin H, et al. Clinical Correlates of Insulin Resistance in Chronic Schizophrenia: Relationship to Negative Symptoms. *Front Psychiatry.* 2019;10:251. Published 2019 Apr 23. doi:10.3389/fpsyt.2019.00251.

16. Gray SM, Meijer RI, Barrett EJ. Insulin regulates brain function, but how does it get there?. *Diabetes.* 2014;63(12):3992-3997. doi:10.2337/db14-0340.

17. National Institutes of Health (US); Biological Sciences Curriculum Study. NIH Curriculum Supplement Series [Internet]. Bethesda (MD): National Institutes of Health (US); 2007. Information about Mental Illness and the Brain. Available from: https://www.ncbi.nlm.nih.gov/books/NBK20369/

18. Knüppel A, Shipley MJ, Llewellyn CH, Brunner EJ. Sugar intake from sweet food and beverages, common mental disorder and depression: prospective findings from the Whitehall II study. *Sci Rep.* 2017;7(1):6287. Published 2017 Jul 27. doi:10.1038/s41598-017-05649-7.

19 Neal, Elizabeth G, et al. "The Ketogenic Diet for the Treatment of Childhood Epilepsy: A Randomized Controlled Trial." *The Lancet Neurology,* Elsevier, 2 May 2008, www.sciencedirect.com/science/article/abs/pii/S1474442208700929.

20. Sirven, Joseph, et al. "The Ketogenic Diet for Intractable Epilepsy in Adults: Preliminary Results." *Wiley Online Library,* John

Wiley & Sons, Ltd, 2 Aug. 2005, onlinelibrary.wiley.com/doi/abs/10.1111/j.1528-1157.1999.tb01589.x.

21.   Lefevre, Frank, and Naomi Aronson. "Ketogenic Diet for the Treatment of Refractory Epilepsy in Children: A Systematic Review of Efficacy." *American Academy of Pediatrics*, American Academy of Pediatrics, 1 Apr. 2000, pediatrics.aappublications.org/content/105/4/e46.

22.   Huttenlocher, P. Ketonemia and Seizures: Metabolic and Anticonvulsant Effects of Two Ketogenic Diets in Childhood Epilepsy. *Pediatr Res* **10,** 536–540 (1976).

23.   Bentley, Jeanie. "International Food Security Assessment, 2020-30." *USDA ERS - Home*, Jan. 2017, www.ers.usda.gov/.

24.   *Diabetes Data and Statistics.* 30 May 2019, www.cdc.gov/diabetes/data/index.html?CDC_AA_refVal=https%3A%2F%2Fwww.cdc.gov%2Fdiabetes%2Fdata%2Findex.htm.

25.   A.D. Lopez et al., eds., Global Burden of Disease and Risk Factors (New York: Oxford University Press, 2006); and C.J.L. Murray and A.D. Lopez, The Global Burden of Disease: A Comparative Assessment of Mortality and Disability from Diseases, Injuries, and Risk Factors in 1990 and Projected to 2020, vol. 1 (Cambridge, Mass.: Harvard University Press, 1996).

26.   Association, American Diabetes. "Consensus Development Conference on Antipsychotic Drugs and Obesity and Diabetes." *Diabetes Care*, American Diabetes Association, 1 Feb. 2004, care.diabetesjournals.org/content/27/2/596.

27.   Avena NM, Rada P, Hoebel BG. Evidence for sugar addiction: behavioral and neurochemical effects of intermittent, excessive sugar intake. *Neurosci Biobehav Rev.* 2008;32(1):20-39. doi:10.1016/j.neubiorev.2007.04.019.

28.   Blusztajn JK, Slack BE, Mellott TJ. Neuroprotective Actions of Dietary Choline. *Nutrients.* 2017;9(8):815. Published 2017 Jul 28. doi:10.3390/nu9080815.

29.   Silverman JM, Schmeidler J. Outcome age-based prediction of successful cognitive aging by total cholesterol. *Alzheimers Dement.* 2018;14(7):952-960. doi:10.1016/j.jalz.2018.01.009.

30.   Berger M, Gray JA, Roth BL. The expanded biology of serotonin. *Annu Rev Med.* 2009;60:355-366. doi:10.1146/annurev.med.60.042307.110802.

31.   Conrad, Brian. "The Role of Dopamine as a Neurotransmitter in the Human Brain." *Enzo Life Sciences*, 2 July 2020, www.enzolifesciences.com/science-center/technotes/2018/november/the-role-of-dopamine-as-a-neurotransmitter-in-the-human-brain/.

Chapter 3: Eating Disorders

1. Wiss D.A., Waterhous T.S. (2014) Nutrition Therapy for Eating Disorders, Substance Use Disorders, and Addictions. In: Brewerton T., Baker Dennis A. (eds) Eating Disorders, Addictions and Substance Use Disorders. Springer, Berlin, Heidelberg. https://doi.org/10.1007/978-3-642-45378-6_23.
2. National Collaborating Centre for Mental Health (UK). Eating Disorders: Core Interventions in the Treatment and Management of Anorexia Nervosa, Bulimia Nervosa and Related Eating Disorders. Leicester (UK): British Psychological Society (UK); 2004. (NICE Clinical Guidelines, No. 9.) 2, Eating disorders. Available from: https://www.ncbi.nlm.nih.gov/books/NBK49318/.
3. Spettigue W, Henderson KA. Eating disorders and the role of the media. *Can Child Adolesc Psychiatr Rev.* 2004;13(1):16-19.
4. Herzog, David B., et al. "Psychiatric Comorbidity in Treatment-Seeking Anorexics and Bulimics." *Journal of the American Academy of Child & Adolescent Psychiatry*, Elsevier, 4 Jan. 2010, www.sciencedirect.com/science/article/abs/pii/S0890856709649637.
5. Braun DL, Sunday SR, Halmi KA. Psychiatric comorbidity in patients with eating disorders. *Psychol Med.* 1994;24(4):859-867. doi:10.1017/s0033291700028956
6. Hudson JI, Hiripi E, Pope HG Jr, Kessler RC. The prevalence and correlates of eating disorders in the National Comorbidity Survey Replication [published correction appears in Biol Psychiatry. 2012 Jul 15;72(2):164]. *Biol Psychiatry.* 2007;61(3):348-358. doi:10.1016/j.biopsych.2006.03.040.
7. Le Grange D, Swanson SA, Crow SJ, Merikangas KR. Eating disorder not otherwise specified presentation in the US population. *Int J Eat Disord.* 2012;45(5):711-718. doi:10.1002/eat.22006.
8. Strother E, Lemberg R, Stanford SC, Turberville D. Eating disorders in men: underdiagnosed, undertreated, and misunderstood. *Eat Disord.* 2012;20(5):346-355. doi:10.1080/10640266.2012.715512.
9. Culbert KM, Racine SE, Klump KL. Research Review: What we have learned about the causes of eating disorders - a synthesis of sociocultural, psychological, and biological research. *J Child Psychol Psychiatry.* 2015;56(11):1141-1164. doi:10.1111/jcpp.12441.
10. "Eating Disorder Statistics • National Association of Anorexia Nervosa and Associated Disorders." *National Association of Anorexia Nervosa and Associated Disorders*, 17 June 2019,

anad.org/education-and-awareness/about-eating-disorders/
eating-disorders-statistics/.

11. Grumet, Karen. "The Role of the Registered Dietitian/Nutritionist on the Eating Disorder Team." *Eating Disorders Catalogue*, 19 Nov. 2014, www.edcatalogue.com/role-registered-dietitian-nutritionist-eating-disorder-team-2/

12. Goldsmith, Toby D. "Bulimia: Binging and Purging." *Psych Central*, 14 Jan. 2020, psychcentral.com/lib/bulimia-binging-and-purging/.

13. "Eating Disorder Statistics • National Association of Anorexia Nervosa and Associated Disorders." *National Association of Anorexia Nervosa and Associated Disorders*, 17 June 2019, anad.org/education-and-awareness/about-eating-disorders/eating-disorders-statistics/.

14. Maino Vieytes CA, Taha HM, Burton-Obanla AA, Douglas KG, Arthur AE. Carbohydrate Nutrition and the Risk of Cancer. Curr Nutr Rep. 2019 Sep;8(3):230-239

15. Belinda Lennerz, Jochen K Lennerz, Food Addiction, High-Glycemic-Index Carbohydrates, and Obesity, *Clinical Chemistry*, Volume 64, Issue 1, 1 January 2018, Pages 64–71, https://doi.org/10.1373/clinchem.2017.273532

16. Geiselman PJ, Novin D. The role of carbohydrates in appetite, hunger and obesity. *Appetite*. 1982;3(3):203-223. doi:10.1016/s0195-6663(82)80017-2

17. Singh M. Mood, food, and obesity. *Front Psychol*. 2014;5:925. Published 2014 Sep 1. doi:10.3389/fpsyg.2014.00925.

18. Keel PK, Dorer DJ, Eddy KT, Franko D, Charatan DL, Herzog DB. Predictors of mortality in eating disorders. *Arch Gen Psychiatry*. 2003;60(2):179-183. doi:10.1001/archpsyc.60.2.179.

19. Portzky G, van Heeringen K, Vervaet M. Attempted suicide in patients with eating disorders. *Crisis*. 2014;35(6):378-387. doi:10.1027/0227-5910/a000275.

20. Patton GC. Mortality in eating disorders. *Psychol Med*. 1988;18(4):947-951. doi:10.1017/s0033291700009879.

21. Arcelus J, Mitchell AJ, Wales J, Nielsen S. Mortality Rates in Patients With Anorexia Nervosa and Other Eating Disorders: A Meta-analysis of 36 Studies. *Arch Gen Psychiatry*. 2011;68(7): 724–731. doi:10.1001/archgenpsychiatry.2011.74.

22. Nowak G, Ordway GA, Paul IA. Alterations in the N-methyl-D-aspartate (NMDA) receptor complex in the frontal cortex of suicide victims. *Brain Res*. 1995;675(1-2):157-164. doi:10.1016/0006-8993(95)00057-w.

23. Holemans S, De Paermentier F, Horton RW, Crompton MR, Katona CL, Maloteaux JM. NMDA glutamatergic receptors, labelled with [3H]MK-801, in brain samples from drug-free depressed suicides. *Brain Res.* 1993;616(1-2):138-143. doi:10.1016/0006-8993(93)90202-x.

24. Berends T, van Meijel B, Nugteren W, et al. Rate, timing and predictors of relapse in patients with anorexia nervosa following a relapse prevention program: a cohort study. *BMC Psychiatry.* 2016;16(1):316. Published 2016 Sep 8. doi:10.1186/s12888-016-1019-y.

25. Kalivas PW. Cocaine and amphetamine-like psychostimulants: neurocircuitry and glutamate neuroplasticity. *Dialogues Clin Neurosci.* 2007;9(4):389-397.

26. Petrilli MA, Kranz TM, Kleinhaus K, et al. The Emerging Role for Zinc in Depression and Psychosis. *Front Pharmacol.* 2017;8:414. Published 2017 Jun 30. doi:10.3389/fphar.2017.00414.

27 Prakash A, Bharti K, Majeed AB. Zinc: indications in brain disorders. *Fundam Clin Pharmacol.* 2015;29(2):131-149. doi:10.1111/fcp.12110.

28. Paoletti P, Ascher P, Neyton J. High-affinity zinc inhibition of NMDA NR1-NR2A receptors [published correction appears in J Neurosci 1997 Oct 15;17(20):followi]. *J Neurosci.* 1997;17(15):5711-5725. doi:10.1523/JNEUROSCI.17-15-05711.1997.

Chapter 4: Sarcopenia

1. Pedersen BK. Muscle as a secretory organ. *Compr Physiol.* 2013;3(3):1337-1362. doi:10.1002/cphy.c120033.

2. Evans W. Functional and metabolic consequences of sarcopenia. *J Nutr.* 1997;127(5 Suppl):998S-1003S. doi:10.1093/jn/127.5.998S.

3. Landi F, Cruz-Jentoft AJ, Liperoti R, et al. Sarcopenia and mortality risk in frail older persons aged 80 years and older: results from ilSIRENTE study. *Age Ageing.* 2013;42(2):203-209. doi:10.1093/ageing/afs194.

4. Bouchonville MF, Villareal DT. Sarcopenic obesity: how do we treat it?. *Curr Opin Endocrinol Diabetes Obes.* 2013;20(5):412-419. doi:10.1097/01.med.0000433071.11466.7f.

5. von Haehling S, Morley JE, Anker SD. An overview of sarcopenia: facts and numbers on prevalence and clinical impact. *J Cachexia Sarcopenia Muscle.* 2010;1(2):129-133. doi:10.1007/s13539-010-0014-2.

6. Morley JE, Argiles JM, Evans WJ, et al. Nutritional recommendations for the management of sarcopenia. *J Am Med Dir Assoc.* 2010;11(6):391-396. doi:10.1016/j.jamda.2010.04.014.

7. Lim S, Kim JH, Yoon JW, et al. Sarcopenic obesity: prevalence and association with metabolic syndrome in the Korean Longitudinal Study on Health and Aging (KLoSHA). *Diabetes Care.* 2010;33(7):1652-1654. doi:10.2337/dc10-0107.

8. Zamboni M, Mazzali G, Zoico E, et al. Health consequences of obesity in the elderly: a review of four unresolved questions. *Int J Obes (Lond).* 2005;29(9):1011-1029. doi:10.1038/sj.ijo.0803005.

9. Berry SD, Samelson EJ, Bordes M, Broe K, Kiel DP. Survival of aged nursing home residents with hip fracture. *J Gerontol A Biol Sci Med Sci.* 2009;64(7):771-777. doi:10.1093/gerona/glp019.

10. von Friesendorff M, Besjakov J, Akesson K. Long-term survival and fracture risk after hip fracture: a 22-year follow-up in women. *J Bone Miner Res.* 2008;23(11):1832-1841. doi:10.1359/jbmr.080606.

11. Rapp K, Becker C, Lamb SE, Icks A, Klenk J. Hip fractures in institutionalized elderly people: incidence rates and excess mortality. *J Bone Miner Res.* 2008;23(11):1825-1831. doi:10.1359/jbmr.080702.

12. Haentjens, P., et al. "Survival and Functional Outcome According to Hip Fracture Type: A One-Year Prospective Cohort Study in Elderly Women with an Intertrochanteric or Femoral Neck Fracture." *Bone*, Elsevier, 30 Aug. 2007, www.sciencedirect.com/science/article/abs/pii/S8756328207006631.

13. Wehren LE, Hawkes WG, Orwig DL, Hebel JR, Zimmerman SI, Magaziner J. Gender differences in mortality after hip fracture: the role of infection. *J Bone Miner Res.* 2003;18(12):2231-2237. doi:10.1359/jbmr.2003.18.12.2231.

14. Richmond J, Aharonoff GB, Zuckerman JD, Koval KJ. Mortality risk after hip fracture. *J Orthop Trauma.* 2003;17(1):53-56. doi:10.1097/00005131-200301000-00008.

15. Elliott J, Beringer T, Kee F, Marsh D, Willis C, Stevenson M. Predicting survival after treatment for fracture of the proximal femur and the effect of delays to surgery. *J Clin Epidemiol.* 2003;56(8):788-795. doi:10.1016/s0895-4356(03)00129-x.

16. Leibson CL, Tosteson AN, Gabriel SE, Ransom JE, Melton LJ. Mortality, disability, and nursing home use for persons with and without hip fracture: a population-based study. *J Am Geriatr Soc.* 2002;50(10):1644-1650. doi:10.1046/j.1532-5415.2002.50455.x.

17. Keene GS, Parker MJ, Pryor GA. Mortality and morbidity after hip fractures. *BMJ*. 1993;307(6914):1248-1250. doi:10.1136/bmj.307.6914.1248.

18. Abrahamsen B, van Staa T, Ariely R, Olson M, Cooper C. Excess mortality following hip fracture: a systematic epidemiological review. *Osteoporos Int*. 2009;20(10):1633-1650. doi:10.1007/s00198-009-0920-3.

19. Friedland, Robert B. "Selected Long-Term Care Statistics." *Selected Long-Term Care Statistics | Family Caregiver Alliance*, 31 Jan. 2015, www.caregiver.org/selected-long-term-care-statistics.

20. Olfson M, Pincus HA. Outpatient mental health care in nonhospital settings: distribution of patients across provider groups. *Am J Psychiatry*. 1996;153(10):1353-1356. doi:10.1176/ajp.153.10.1353.

21. Rao TS, Asha MR, Ramesh BN, Rao KS. Understanding nutrition, depression and mental illnesses. *Indian J Psychiatry*. 2008;50(2):77-82. doi:10.4103/0019-5545.42391.

22. Houston DK, Nicklas BJ, Ding J, et al. Dietary protein intake is associated with lean mass change in older, community-dwelling adults: the Health, Aging, and Body Composition (Health ABC) Study. *Am J Clin Nutr*. 2008;87(1):150-155. doi:10.1093/ajcn/87.1.150.

23. Nowson C, O'Connell S. Protein Requirements and Recommendations for Older People: A Review. *Nutrients*. 2015;7(8):6874-6899. Published 2015 Aug 14. doi:10.3390/nu7085311.

24. Wolfe RR, Miller SL. The recommended dietary allowance of protein: a misunderstood concept [published correction appears in JAMA. 2008 Oct 15;300(15):1763]. *JAMA*. 2008;299(24):2891-2893. doi:10.1001/jama.299.24.2891.

25. Bunker, V., Lawson, M., Stansfield, M., & Clayton, B. (1987). Nitrogen balance studies in apparently healthy elderly people and those who are housebound. British Journal of Nutrition, 57(2), 211-221. Doi:10.1079/BJN19870027.

26. Pepersack T, Corretge M, Beyer I, et al. Examining the effect of intervention to nutritional problems of hospitalised elderly: a pilot project. *J Nutr Health Aging*. 2002;6(5):306-310.

27. Bellanger TM, Bray GA. Obesity related morbidity and mortality. *J La State Med Soc*. 2005;157 Spec No 1:S42-49.

28. Klein S, Burke LE, Bray GA, et al. Clinical implications of obesity with specific focus on cardiovascular disease: a statement for professionals from the American Heart Association Council on Nutrition, Physical Activity, and Metabolism: endorsed by the American College of Cardiology Foundation. *Circulation*. 2004;110(18):2952-2967. doi:10.1161/01.CIR.0000145546.97738.1E.

29. Glynn EL, Fry CS, Drummond MJ, et al. Excess leucine intake enhances muscle anabolic signaling but not net protein anabolism in young men and women. *J Nutr.* 2010;140(11):1970-1976. doi:10.3945/jn.110.127647.

30. Breen L, Phillips SM. Skeletal muscle protein metabolism in the elderly: Interventions to counteract the 'anabolic resistance' of ageing. *Nutr Metab (Lond).* 2011;8:68. Published 2011 Oct 5. doi:10.1186/1743-7075-8-68.

31. Paddon-Jones D, Sheffield-Moore M, Zhang XJ, et al. Amino acid ingestion improves muscle protein synthesis in the young and elderly. *Am J Physiol Endocrinol Metab.* 2004;286(3):E321-E328. doi:10.1152/ajpendo.00368.2003.

32. Rand WM, Pellett PL, Young VR. Meta-analysis of nitrogen balance studies for estimating protein requirements in healthy adults. *Am J Clin Nutr.* 2003;77(1):109-127. doi:10.1093/ajcn/77.1.109.

33. Schlemmer U, Frølich W, Prieto RM, Grases F. Phytate in foods and significance for humans: food sources, intake, processing, bioavailability, protective role and analysis. *Mol Nutr Food Res.* 2009;53 Suppl 2:S330-S375. doi:10.1002/mnfr.200900099.

34. Institute of Medicine (US) Food Forum. Providing Healthy and Safe Foods As We Age: Workshop Summary. Washington (DC): National Academies Press (US); 2010. Available from: https://www.ncbi.nlm.nih.gov/books/NBK51847/ doi: 10.17226/12967.

35. "How Much Physical Activity Do Older Adults Need?" *Centers for Disease Control and Prevention*, Centers for Disease Control and Prevention, 9 Oct. 2020, www.cdc.gov/physicalactivity/basics/older_adults/index.htm.

Chapter 5: Heart Disease

1. Heron, Melanie. "National Vital Statistics Report." *Deaths: Leading Causes for 2017*, CDC, 24 June 2019, www.cdc.gov/nchs/data/nvsr/nvsr68/nvsr68_06-508.pdf

2. Benjamin EJ, Muntner P, Alonso A, Bittencourt MS, Callaway CW, Carson AP, et al. Heart disease and stroke statistics—2019 update: a report from the American Heart Association. *Circulation.* 2019;139(10):e56–528.

3. Lisa Brown, Bernard Rosner, Walter W Willett, Frank M Sacks, Cholesterol-lowering effects of dietary fiber: a meta-analysis, *The*

American Journal of Clinical Nutrition, Volume 69, Issue 1, January 1999, Pages 30–42, https://doi.org/10.1093/ajcn/69.1.30

4. Zampelas A, Magriplis E. New Insights into Cholesterol Functions: A Friend or an Enemy?. *Nutrients*. 2019;11(7):1645. Published 2019 Jul 18. doi:10.3390/nu11071645.

5. Strott CA, Higashi Y. Cholesterol sulfate in human physiology: what's it all about?. *J Lipid Res*. 2003;44(7):1268-1278. doi:10.1194/jlr. R300005-JLR200.

6. Netea MG, Demacker PN, Kullberg BJ, et al. Low-density lipoprotein receptor-deficient mice are protected against lethal endotoxemia and severe gram-negative infections. *J Clin Invest*. 1996;97(6):1366-1372. doi:10.1172/JCI118556.

7. de Bont N, Netea MG, Demacker PN, et al. Apolipoprotein E knockout mice are highly susceptible to endotoxemia and Klebsiella pneumoniae infection. *J Lipid Res*. 1999;40(4):680-685.

8. Fan J, Wang H, Ye G, et al. Letter to the Editor: Low-density lipoprotein is a potential predictor of poor prognosis in patients with coronavirus disease 2019. *Metabolism*. 2020;107:154243. doi:10.1016/j.metabol.2020.154243.

9. Huggins, Siobhan. "Lipoprotein Power – LDL and the Immune System." *Cholesterol Code*, Cholesterol Code, 21 June 2019, cholesterolcode.com/lipoprotein-power-ldl-and-the-immune-system/.

10. Simonnet, A., et al., *High Prevalence of Obesity in Severe Acute Respiratory Syndrome Coronavirus-2 (SARS-CoV-2) Requiring Invasive Mechanical Ventilation*. Obesity (Silver Spring), 2020.

11. Kalligeros, M., et al., *Association of Obesity with Disease Severity Among Patients with Coronavirus Disease 2019*. Obesity, 2020(n/a).

12. Weverling-Rijnsburger AW, Blauw GJ, Lagaay AM, Knook DL, Meinders AE, Westendorp RG. Total cholesterol and risk of mortality in the oldest old [published correction appears in Lancet 1998 Jan 3;351(9095):70]. *Lancet*. 1997;350(9085):1119-1123. doi:10.1016/s0140-6736(97)04430-9.

13. Jacobs D, Blackburn H, Higgins M, et al. Report of the Conference on Low Blood Cholesterol: Mortality Associations. *Circulation*. 1992;86(3):1046-1060. doi:10.1161/01.cir.86.3.1046.

14. Neaton JD, Wentworth DN. Low serum cholesterol and risk of death from AIDS. *AIDS*. 1997;11(7):929-930.

15. Soliman GA. Dietary Cholesterol and the Lack of Evidence in Cardiovascular Disease. *Nutrients*. 2018;10(6):780. Published 2018 Jun 16. doi:10.3390/nu10060780.

16. Iribarren C, Jacobs DR Jr, Sidney S, Claxton AJ, Feingold KR. Cohort study of serum total cholesterol and in-hospital incidence of infectious diseases. *Epidemiol Infect*. 1998;121(2):335-347. doi:10.1017/s0950268898001435.

17. Chowdhury R, Warnakula S, Kunutsor S, et al. Association of dietary, circulating, and supplement fatty acids with coronary risk: a systematic review and meta-analysis [published correction appears in Ann Intern Med. 2014 May 6;160(9):658]. *Ann Intern Med*. 2014;160(6):398-406. doi:10.7326/M13-1788.

18. Olsson U, Egnell AC, Lee MR, et al. Changes in matrix proteoglycans induced by insulin and fatty acids in hepatic cells may contribute to dyslipidemia of insulin resistance. *Diabetes*. 2001;50(9):2126-2132. doi:10.2337/diabetes.50.9.2126.

19. Hulthe J, Bokemark L, Wikstrand J, Fagerberg B. The metabolic syndrome, LDL particle size, and atherosclerosis: the Atherosclerosis and Insulin Resistance (AIR) study. *Arterioscler Thromb Vasc Biol*. 2000;20(9):2140-2147. doi:10.1161/01.atv.20.9.2140.

20. Wasty, F., Alavi, M.Z. & Moore, S. Distribution of glycosaminoglycans in the intima of human aortas: changes in atherosclerosis and diabetes mellitus. *Diabetologia* **36,** 316–322 (1993). https://doi.org/10.1007/BF00400234

21. Rodriguéz-Lee, Mariama; Bondjers, Görana,b; Camejo, Germána,c Fatty acid-induced atherogenic changes in extracellular matrix proteoglycans, Current Opinion in Lipidology: October 2007 - Volume 18 - Issue 5 - p 546-553 doi: 10.1097/MOL.0b013e3282ef534f.

22. Ulijaszek, Stanley J., et al., 1991 Human Dietary Change. Philosophical Transactions: Biological Sciences, 334 (1270): 271-279.

23. Eastman, Richard C, and Harry Keen. "The Impact of Cardiovascular Disease on People with Diabetes: The Potential for Prevention." The Lancet, July 1997, doi.org/10.1016/S0140-6736(97)90026-X.

24. SALADINO, PAUL. *CARNIVORE CODE: Unlocking the Secrets to Optimal Health by Returning to Our Ancestral Diet*. HOUGHTON MIFFLIN HARCOURT, 2020.

25. O'Connor, Anahad. "How the Sugar Industry Shifted Blame to Fat." *New York Times*, 13 Sept. 2016, p. 1., doi:https://www.nytimes.com/2016/09/13/well/eat/how-the-sugar-industry-shifted-blame-to-fat.html.

26. Holland, Kimberly. "Paleo and Keto Diets May Hurt Your Heart." *Healthline*, Healthline Media, 30 July 2019, www.healthline.com/health-news/paleo-keto-diet-may-increase-your-risk-for-heart-disease

27. Velasquez MT, Ramezani A, Manal A, Raj DS. Trimethylamine N-Oxide: The Good, the Bad and the Unknown. *Toxins (Basel)*. 2016;8(11):326. Published 2016 Nov 8. doi:10.3390/toxins8110326.
28. Zeisel SH, da Costa KA. Choline: an essential nutrient for public health. *Nutr Rev*. 2009;67(11):615-623. doi:10.1111/j.1753-4887.2009.00246.x
29. Alesci, S., Manoli, I., Costello, R., Coates, P., Gold, P. W., Chrousos, G. P., & Blackman, M. R. (2004). Carnitine: Lessons from one hundred years of research. *Annals of the New York Academy of Sciences, 1033*, ix-xi. https://doi.org/10.1196/annals.1320.019.
30. Dambrova M, Latkovskis G, Kuka J, et al. Diabetes is Associated with Higher Trimethylamine N-oxide Plasma Levels. *Exp Clin Endocrinol Diabetes*. 2016;124(4):251-256. doi:10.1055/s-0035-1569330.
31. Janeiro MH, Ramírez MJ, Milagro FI, Martínez JA, Solas M. Implication of Trimethylamine N-Oxide (TMAO) in Disease: Potential Biomarker or New Therapeutic Target. *Nutrients*. 2018;10(10):1398. Published 2018 Oct 1. doi:10.3390/nu10101398.
32. Cheung W, Keski-Rahkonen P, Assi N, et al. A metabolomic study of biomarkers of meat and fish intake. *Am J Clin Nutr*. 2017;105(3): 600-608. doi:10.3945/ajcn.116.146639.
33. Jia J, Dou P, Gao M, et al. Assessment of Causal Direction Between Gut Microbiota-Dependent Metabolites and Cardiometabolic Health: A Bidirectional Mendelian Randomization Analysis. *Diabetes*. 2019;68(9):1747-1755. doi:10.2337/db19-0153.
34. Sergio López, Beatriz Bermúdez, Yolanda M Pacheco, José Villar, Rocío Abia, Francisco JG Muriana, Distinctive postprandial modulation of β cell function and insulin sensitivity by dietary fats: monounsaturated compared with saturated fatty acids, *The American Journal of Clinical Nutrition*, Volume 88, Issue 3, September 2008, Pages 638–644, https://doi.org/10.1093/ajcn/88.3.638.

Chapter 6: Where the F Did the Nutrition Guidelines come from?

1. (1986, April). *Ministry Magazine Ellen G White and Vegetarianism*. doi:https://www.ministrymagazine.org/archive/1986/06/
2. White, E. (n.d.). *Ministry Magazine Testimony Studies on Diets and Foods*, 20.
3. White, E. G. (1864). *An Appeal to Mothers*.
4. Risley, E., Dr. (1922). The Newer Dietetics. *Loma Linda University Publications The Medical Evangelist, 8*(6). doi:https://

scholarsrepository.llu.edu/cgi/viewcontent.cgi?article=1044&-context=medical_evangelist

5. Training School for Dietitians—A New Course of Study at Loma Linda. (1922). *Loma Linda University Publications The Medical Evangelist, 9*(1), 24-25.

6. Vegetarians and Vitamin B12: An interview with Mervyn G. Hardinge, M.D., Dr.P.H., Ph.D. (1983). *Your Life or Your Health,* 14-15.

7. Melina V, Craig W, Levin S. Position of the Academy of Nutrition and Dietetics: Vegetarian Diets. J Acad Nutr Diet. 2016 Dec;116(12):1970-1980. doi: 10.1016/j.jand.2016.09.025. PMID: 27886704.

8. White, J., & White, E. (1890). *Christian temperance and bible hygiene*. Michigan.

9. Malhotra A, Redberg RF, Meier P Saturated fat does not clog the arteries: coronary heart disease is a chronic inflammatory condition, the risk of which can be effectively reduced from healthy lifestyle interventions *British Journal of Sports Medicine* 2017;51: 1111-1112.

10. Soliman, G. (2018, June 16). Dietary Cholesterol and the Lack of Evidence in Cardiovascular Disease. Retrieved November 18, 2020, from https://www.ncbi.nlm.nih.gov/pmc/articles/PMC6024687/

11. Rosch PJ. Cholesterol does not cause coronary heart disease in contrast to stress. Scand Cardiovasc J. 2008 Aug;42(4):244-9. doi: 10.1080/14017430801993701. PMID: 18609060.

12. Domonoske, C. (2016, September 13). 50 Years Ago, Sugar Industry Quietly Paid Scientists To Point Blame At Fat. Retrieved November 18, 2020, from https://www.npr.org/sections/thetwo-way/2016/09/13/493739074/50-years-ago-sugar-industry-quietly-paid-scientists-to-point-blame-at-fat

13. Farming in the 1940's Food For War. (n.d.). Retrieved November 18, 2020, from https://livinghistoryfarm.org/farminginthe40s/money_02.html

14. Peretti, J. (2012, June 11). Why our food is making us fat. Retrieved November 18, 2020, from https://www.theguardian.com/business/2012/jun/11/why-our-food-is-making-us-fat

15. Anson, R. S. (1972). *McGovern: A Biography* (pp. 218-242). New York: Holt, Rinehart and Winston.

16. Oppenheimer GM, Benrubi ID. McGovern's Senate Select Committee on Nutrition and Human Needs versus the meat industry on the diet-heart question (1976-1977). *Am J Public Health.* 2014;104(1):59-69. doi:10.2105/AJPH.2013.301464

17.   Dietary Goals for the United States. (1977). Retrieved from https://catalog.princeton.edu/catalog/1237598

18.   Oppenheimer, Gerald Benrubi, I 2013/11/14 T1 - McGovern's Senate Select Committee on Nutrition and Human Needs Versus the: Meat Industry on the Diet-Heart Question (1976–1977) VL - 104 DO - 10.2105/AJPH.2013.301464 JO - American journal of public health

19.   Let's Remember What SNAP Is For. (2017, October 11). Retrieved November 18, 2020, from https://www.cbpp.org/blog/lets-remember-what-snap-is-for

20.   Testimony of Robert Greenstein, President, Center on Budget and Policy Priorities Before the House Committee on Agriculture. (2017, October 11). Retrieved November 18, 2020, from https://www.cbpp.org/testimony-of-robert-greenstein-president-center-on-budget-and-policy-priorities-before-the-house

21.   Eisinger, P. K. (1998). *Toward an end to hunger in America* (pp. 78-85). Washington, DC: Brookings Inst. Press.

22.   Nestle, M. (2007). *Food Politics: How the Food Industry Influences Nutrition and Health (2nd ed.)* (pp. 38-42). University of California Press.

23.   Soliman, G. (2018, June 16). Dietary Cholesterol and the Lack of Evidence in Cardiovascular Disease. Retrieved November 18, 2020, from https://www.ncbi.nlm.nih.gov/pmc/articles/PMC6024687/

24.   Ending the War on Fat. (2014, June 12). Retrieved November 18, 2020, from https://time.com/magazine/us/2863200/june-23rd-2014-vol-183-no-24-u-s/

25.   Ifland JR, Preuss HG, Marcus MT, Rourke KM, Taylor WC, Burau K, Jacobs WS, Kadish W, Manso G. Refined food addiction: a classic substance use disorder. Med Hypotheses. 2009 May;72(5):518-26. doi: 10.1016/j.mehy.2008.11.035. Epub 2009 Feb 14. PMID: 19223127.

26.   Spring B, Schneider K, Smith M, Kendzor D, Appelhans B, Hedeker D, Pagoto S. Abuse potential of carbohydrates for overweight carbohydrate cravers. Psychopharmacology (Berl). 2008 May;197(4):637-47. doi: 10.1007/s00213-008-1085-z. Epub 2008 Feb 14. PMID: 18273603; PMCID: PMC2829437.

27.   Cocores JA, Gold MS. The Salted Food Addiction Hypothesis may explain overeating and the obesity epidemic. Med Hypotheses. 2009 Dec;73(6):892-9. doi: 10.1016/j.mehy.2009.06.049. Epub 2009 Jul 29. PMID: 19643550.

28.   Gearhardt AN, Davis C, Kuschner R, Brownell KD. The addiction potential of hyperpalatable foods. Curr Drug Abuse Rev. 2011 Sep;4(3): 140-5. doi: 10.2174/1874473711104030140. PMID: 21999688.

29. Aktas G, Alcelik A, Yalcin A, et al. Treatment of iron deficiency anemia induces weight loss and improves metabolic parameters. La Clinica Terapeutica. 2014 Mar-Apr;165(2):e87-9. DOI: 10.7471/ct.2014.1688.

30. Simon, M. (2013, January). Are America's Nutrition Professionals in the Pocket of Big Food? Retrieved from https://www.eatdrinkpolitics.com/wp-content/uploads/AND_Corporate_Sponsorship_Report.pdf

31. O'Connor, A. (2015, September 28). Coke Spends Lavishly on Pediatricians and Dietitians. Retrieved November 18, 2020, from https://well.blogs.nytimes.com/2015/09/28/coke-spends-lavishly-on-pediatricians-and-dietitians/

32. Kapell, M., & McVeigh, S. (2011). *The films of James Cameron critical essays*. Jefferson, NC: McFarland &.

33. Casinader, J. (2019, June 16). Sir Peter Jackson and James Cameron team up to promote meatless future. Retrieved November 18, 2020, from https://web.archive.org/web/20190928151333/https://www.stuff.co.nz/business/113246523/sir-peter-jackson-and-james-cameron-team-up-to-promote-meatless-future

34. House JK, Smith BP, Fecteau G, VanMetre DC. Assessment of the ruminant digestive system. Vet Clin North Am Food Anim Pract. 1992 Jul;8(2):189-202. doi: 10.1016/s0749-0720(15)30747-7. PMID: 1643556.

35. Marieb, E. N., & Hoehn, K. (2019). *Human anatomy & physiology*. Harlow, Essex: Pearson Education Limited.

36. Beasley DE, Koltz AM, Lambert JE, Fierer N, Dunn RR. The Evolution of Stomach Acidity and Its Relevance to the Human Microbiome. *PLoS One*. 2015;10(7):e0134116. Published 2015 Jul 29. doi:10.1371/journal.pone.0134116

37. Henry, T. (2018, November 26). Adult obesity rates rise in 6 states, exceed 35% in 7. Retrieved November 18, 2020, from https://www.ama-assn.org/delivering-care/public-health/adult-obesity-rates-rise-6-states-exceed-35-7

38. The Seventh-day Adventist Church's Understanding of Ellen White's Authority. (n.d.). Retrieved November 18, 2020, from https://whiteestate.org/legacy/issues-scripsda-html/

39. Anderson, H. A. (2013). *Breakfast: A history*. Lanham, MD: Altamira Press.

40. Buckley, N. (2020, January 09). How John Harvey Kellogg was wrong on race. Retrieved November 18, 2020, from https://www.battlecreekenquirer.com/story/news/2019/03/21/john-harvey-kellogg-battle-creek-michigan-eugenics-race-nazis/3202628002/

41. Leung, C. (n.d.). Kellogg, John Harvey. Retrieved November 18, 2020, from http://eugenicsarchive.ca/discover/connections/512fa0d334c5399e2c00

42. Sorokie, A. M. (2008). *Gut wisdom: Understanding and improving your digestive health.* Sydney, Australia: ReadHowYouWant.

43. Mawdsley, E. (2020, July 08). America and WW2: When, how and why did the US get involved, and why they didn't enter sooner? Retrieved November 18, 2020, from https://www.historyextra.com/period/second-world-war/why-when-how-america-entered-ww2-pearl-harbor-roosevelt/

44. Johnston BC, Zeraatkar D, Han MA, Vernooij RWM, Valli C, El Dib R, Marshall C, Stover PJ, Fairweather-Taitt S, Wójcik G, Bhatia F, de Souza R, Brotons C, Meerpohl JJ, Patel CJ, Djulbegovic B, Alonso-Coello P, Bala MM, Guyatt GH. Unprocessed Red Meat and Processed Meat Consumption: Dietary Guideline Recommendations From the Nutritional Recommendations (NutriRECS) Consortium. Ann Intern Med. 2019 Nov 19;171(10):756-764. doi: 10.7326/M19-1621. Epub 2019 Oct 1. PMID: 31569235.

45. RODGERS, DIANA WOLF ROBB. *SACRED COW.* BENBELLA Books, 2020.

Chapter 7: Plants vs Animals

1. Widad Makhdour Al-Bishri, Enas Nabil Danial and Nadia Ameen Abdelmajeed, 2018. Reducing Osteoporosis by Phytase Supplemented Diet in Albino Rats. *International Journal of Pharmacology, 14: 121-126.*

2. Vasconcelos IM, Oliveira JT. Antinutritional properties of plant lectins. Toxicon. 2004 Sep 15;44(4):385-403. doi: 10.1016/j.toxicon.2004.05.005. PMID: 15302522.

3. Kong S, Zhang YH, Zhang W. Regulation of Intestinal Epithelial Cells Properties and Functions by Amino Acids. Biomed Res Int. 2018 May 9;2018:2819154. doi: 10.1155/2018/2819154. PMID: 29854738; PMCID: PMC5966675.

4. Kong, S., Zhang, Y., & Zhang, W. (2018, May 09). Regulation of Intestinal Epithelial Cells Properties and Functions by Amino Acids. Retrieved from https://www.hindawi.com/journals/bmri/2018/2819154/.

5. Kennedy, Eileen, et al. "The 1995 Dietary Guidelines for Americans: An Overview." *Journal of the American Dietetic Association,*

Elsevier, 24 Apr. 2003, www.sciencedirect.com/science/article/abs/pii/S0002822396000727.

6. Watanabe F, Katsura H, Takenaka S, Fujita T, Abe K, Tamura Y, Nakatsuka T, Nakano Y. Pseudovitamin B(12) is the predominant cobamide of an algal health food, spirulina tablets. J Agric Food Chem. 1999 Nov;47(11):4736-41. doi: 10.1021/jf990541b. PMID: 10552882.

7. Gilsing AM, Crowe FL, Lloyd-Wright Z, Sanders TA, Appleby PN, Allen NE, Key TJ. Serum concentrations of vitamin B12 and folate in British male omnivores, vegetarians and vegans: results from a cross-sectional analysis of the EPIC-Oxford cohort study. Eur J Clin Nutr. 2010 Sep;64(9):933-9. doi: 10.1038/ejcn.2010.142. Epub 2010 Jul 21. PMID: 20648045; PMCID: PMC2933506.

8. Herrmann W, Schorr H, Obeid R, Geisel J. Vitamin B-12 status, particularly holotranscobalamin II and methylmalonic acid concentrations, and hyperhomocysteinemia in vegetarians. Am J Clin Nutr. 2003 Jul;78(1):131-6. doi: 10.1093/ajcn/78.1.131. PMID: 12816782.

9. Lachner C, Steinle NI, Regenold WT. The neuropsychiatry of vitamin B12 deficiency in elderly patients. J Neuropsychiatry Clin Neurosci. 2012 Winter;24(1):5-15. doi: 10.1176/appi.neuropsych.11020052. PMID: 22450609.

10. Tripkovic L, Lambert H, Hart K, et al. Comparison of vitamin D2 and vitamin D3 supplementation in raising serum 25-hydroxyvitamin D status: a systematic review and meta-analysis. *Am J Clin Nutr.* 2012;95(6):1357-1364. doi:10.3945/ajcn.111.031070

11. "Global Anaemia Prevalence and Number of Individuals Affected." *World Health Organization*, World Health Organization, 9 July 2008, www.who.int/vmnis/anaemia/prevalence/summary/anaemia_data_status_t2/en/.

12. Scrimshaw NS. Iron deficiency. Sci Am. 1991 Oct;265(4):46-52. doi: 10.1038/scientificamerican1091-46. Erratum in: Sci Am 1992 Jan;266(1):following 8. PMID: 1745900.

13. Craig WJ. Nutrition concerns and health effects of vegetarian diets. Nutr Clin Pract. 2010 Dec;25(6):613-20. doi: 10.1177/0884533610385707. PMID: 21139125.

14. Weaver CM, Proulx WR, Heaney R. Choices for achieving adequate dietary calcium with a vegetarian diet. Am J Clin Nutr. 1999 Sep;70(3 Suppl):543S-548S. doi: 10.1093/ajcn/70.3.543s. PMID: 10479229.

15. Iguacel I, Miguel-Berges ML, Gómez-Bruton A, Moreno LA, Julián C. Veganism, vegetarianism, bone mineral density, and fracture

risk: a systematic review and meta-analysis. Nutr Rev. 2019 Jan 1;77(1):1-18. doi: 10.1093/nutrit/nuy045. PMID: 30376075.

16. Freeland-Graves JH, Bodzy PW, Eppright MA. Zinc status of vegetarians. J Am Diet Assoc. 1980 Dec;77(6):655-61. PMID: 7440860.

17 Burns-Whitmore B, Froyen E, Heskey C, Parker T, San Pablo G. Alpha-Linolenic and Linoleic Fatty Acids in the Vegan Diet: Do They Require Dietary Reference Intake/Adequate Intake Special Consideration?. *Nutrients*. 2019;11(10):2365. Published 2019 Oct 4. doi:10.3390/nu11102365.

18. Ede, Georgia. "The Brain Needs Animal Fat." *Psychology Today*, Sussex Publishers, 31 Mar. 2019, www.psychologytoday.com/us/blog/diagnosis-diet/201903/the-brain-needs-animal-fat.

19. Cholewski M, Tomczykowa M, Tomczyk M. A Comprehensive Review of Chemistry, Sources and Bioavailability of Omega-3 Fatty Acids. *Nutrients*. 2018;10(11):1662. Published 2018 Nov 4. doi:10.3390/nu10111662

20. Melina V, Craig W, Levin S. Position of the Academy of Nutrition and Dietetics: Vegetarian Diets. J Acad Nutr Diet. 2016 Dec;116(12):1970-1980. doi: 10.1016/j.jand.2016.09.025. PMID: 27886704.

21. Dalla Pellegrina C, Perbellini O, Scupoli MT, Tomelleri C, Zanetti C, Zoccatelli G, Fusi M, Peruffo A, Rizzi C, Chignola R. Effects of wheat germ agglutinin on human gastrointestinal epithelium: insights from an experimental model of immune/epithelial cell interaction. Toxicol Appl Pharmacol. 2009 Jun 1;237(2):146-53. doi: 10.1016/j.taap.2009.03.012. Epub 2009 Mar 28. PMID: 19332085.

22. Bharucha AE, Pemberton JH, Locke GR 3rd. American Gastroenterological Association technical review on constipation. *Gastroenterology*. 2013;144(1):218-238. doi:10.1053/j.gastro.2012.10.028.

23. Bielefeldt K, Levinthal DJ, Nusrat S. Effective Constipation Treatment Changes More Than Bowel Frequency: A Systematic Review and Meta-Analysis. *J Neurogastroenterol Motil*. 2016;22(1):31-45. doi:10.5056/jnm15171.

24. Ho KS, Tan CY, Mohd Daud MA, Seow-Choen F. Stopping or reducing dietary fiber intake reduces constipation and its associated symptoms. *World J Gastroenterol*. 2012;18(33):4593-4596. doi:10.3748/wjg.v18.i33.4593.

25. Weizman AV, Nguyen GC. Diverticular disease: epidemiology and management. *Can J Gastroenterol*. 2011;25(7):385-389. doi:10.1155/2011/795241.

26. Lin OS, Soon MS, Wu SS, Chen YY, Hwang KL, Triadafilopoulos G. Dietary habits and right-sided colonic diverticulosis. Dis Colon Rectum. 2000 Oct;43(10):1412-8. doi: 10.1007/BF02236638. PMID: 11052519.

27. Song JH, Kim YS, Lee JH, et al. Clinical characteristics of colonic diverticulosis in Korea: a prospective study. *Korean J Intern Med.* 2010;25(2):140-146. doi:10.3904/kjim.2010.25.2.140.

28. Torre M, Rodriguez AR, Saura-Calixto F. Effects of dietary fiber and phytic acid on mineral availability. Crit Rev Food Sci Nutr. 1991;30(1):1-22. doi: 10.1080/10408399109527539. PMID: 1657026.

29. Corrigan, Mandy L., et al. *Adult Short Bowel Syndrome: Nutritional, Medical, and Surgical Management.* Elsevier/Academic Press, 2019.

30. So D, Whelan K, Rossi M, Morrison M, Holtmann G, Kelly JT, Shanahan ER, Staudacher HM, Campbell KL. Dietary fiber intervention on gut microbiota composition in healthy adults: a systematic review and meta-analysis. Am J Clin Nutr. 2018 Jun 1;107(6):965-983. doi: 10.1093/ajcn/nqy041. PMID: 29757343.

31. David, L., Maurice, C., Carmody, R. *et al.* Diet rapidly and reproducibly alters the human gut microbiome. *Nature* 505, 559–563 (2014). https://doi.org/10.1038/nature12820

32. Saladino, Paul, and Mark Sisson. *The Carnivore Code.* Houghton Mifflin Harcourt, 2020.

33. Crane TE, Kubota C, West JL, Kroggel MA, Wertheim BC, Thomson CA. Increasing the vegetable intake dose is associated with a rise in plasma carotenoids without modifying oxidative stress or inflammation in overweight or obese postmenopausal women. J Nutr. 2011 Oct;141(10):1827-33. doi: 10.3945/jn.111.139659. Epub 2011 Aug 24. PMID: 21865569; PMCID: PMC3174856.

34. Møller P, Vogel U, Pedersen A, Dragsted LO, Sandström B, Loft S. No effect of 600 grams fruit and vegetables per day on oxidative DNA damage and repair in healthy nonsmokers. Cancer Epidemiol Biomarkers Prev. 2003 Oct;12(10):1016-22. PMID: 14578137.

35. Peluso I, Raguzzini A, Catasta G, Cammisotto V, Perrone A, Tomino C, Toti E, Serafini M. Effects of High Consumption of Vegetables on Clinical, Immunological, and Antioxidant Markers in Subjects at Risk of Cardiovascular Diseases. Oxid Med Cell Longev. 2018 Oct 8;2018:5417165. doi: 10.1155/2018/5417165. PMID: 30402206; PMCID: PMC6196889.

36. Young JF, Dragstedt LO, Haraldsdóttir J, Daneshvar B, Kall MA, Loft S, Nilsson L, Nielsen SE, Mayer B, Skibsted LH, Huynh-Ba T, Hermetter A, Sandström B. Green tea extract only affects markers of oxidative status postprandially: lasting antioxidant effect of flavonoid-free diet. Br J Nutr. 2002 Apr;87(4):343-55. doi: 10.1079/bjn-bjn2002523. PMID: 12064344.

37. Keim, Brandon. "The Surprisingly Complicated Math of How Many Wild Animals Are Killed in Agriculture." *Anthropocene*, July 2018, www.anthropocenemagazine.org/2018/07/how-many-animals-killed-in-agriculture/

38. Morales FE Ms, Tinsley GM, Gordon PM. Acute and Long-Term Impact of High-Protein Diets on Endocrine and Metabolic Function, Body Composition, and Exercise-Induced Adaptations. J Am Coll Nutr. 2017 May-Jun;36(4):295-305. doi: 10.1080/07315724.2016.1274691. Epub 2017 Apr 26. PMID: 28443785.

39. Swift, Roger S. "Sequestration of Carbon by Soil." *Soil science*, v. 166,.11 pp. 858-871. doi: 10.1097/00010694-200111000-00010.

40. Ontl, Todd & Schulte, L.A.. (2012). Soil carbon storage. Nature Education Knowledge. 3.

41. "Sources of Greenhouse Gas Emissions." *EPA*, Environmental Protection Agency, 9 Sept. 2020, www.epa.gov/ghgemissions/sources-greenhouse-gas-emissions.

42. Herbert Wieser, Chemistry of gluten proteins, Food Microbiology, Volume 24, Issue 2, 2007, Pages 115-119, ISSN 0740-0020, https://doi.org/10.1016/j.fm.2006.07.004. (http://www.sciencedirect.com/science/article/pii/S0740002006001535).

43. Cohen IS, Day AS, Shaoul R. Gluten in Celiac Disease-More or Less?. *Rambam Maimonides Med J*. 2019;10(1):e0007. Published 2019 Jan 28. doi:10.5041/RMMJ.10360

44. Lundin KE, Alaedini A. Non-celiac gluten sensitivity. Gastrointest Endosc Clin N Am. 2012 Oct;22(4):723-34. doi: 10.1016/j.giec.2012.07.006. Epub 2012 Aug 17. PMID: 23083989.

45. Ruuskanen A, Luostarinen L, Collin P, Krekela I, Patrikainen H, Tillonen J, et al. Persistently positive gliadin antibodies without transglutaminase antibodies in the elderly: gluten intolerance beyond coeliac disease. *Dig Liver Dis* (2011) **43**(10):772–8. doi:10.1016/j.dld.2011.04.025.

46. Rashtak S, Murray JA. Celiac disease in the elderly. *Gastroenterol Clin North Am*. 2009;38(3):433-446. doi:10.1016/j.gtc.2009.06.005.

47. Dalla Pellegrina C, Perbellini O, Scupoli MT, Tomelleri C, Zanetti C, Zoccatelli G, Fusi M, Peruffo A, Rizzi C, Chignola R. Effects of wheat germ agglutinin on human gastrointestinal epithelium: insights from an experimental model of immune/epithelial cell interaction. Toxicol Appl Pharmacol. 2009 Jun 1;237(2):146-53. doi: 10.1016/j. taap.2009.03.012. Epub 2009 Mar 28. PMID: 19332085.

48. Karlsson A. Wheat germ agglutinin induces NADPH-oxidase activity in human neutrophils by interaction with mobilizable receptors. *Infect Immun*. 1999;67(7):3461-3468. doi:10.1128/IAI.67.7.3461-3468.1999.

49. Zevallos V, Yogev N, Nikolaev A et al. Consumption of wheat alpha-amylase/trypsin inhibitors (ATIs) enhances experimental autoimmune encephalomyelitis in mice. Oral presentation at the 16th International Coeliac Disease Symposium, 21-24 June 2015, Prague, Czech Republic.

50. Junker Y, Zeissig S, Kim SJ, et al. Wheat amylase trypsin inhibitors drive intestinal inflammation via activation of toll-like receptor 4. *J Exp Med*. 2012;209(13):2395-2408. doi:10.1084/jem.20102660.

51. Konstantynowicz J, Porowski T, Zoch-Zwierz W, Wasilewska J, Kadziela-Olech H, Kulak W, Owens SC, Piotrowska-Jastrzebska J, Kaczmarski M. A potential pathogenic role of oxalate in autism. Eur J Paediatr Neurol. 2012 Sep;16(5):485-91. doi: 10.1016/j. ejpn.2011.08.004. Epub 2011 Sep 10. PMID: 21911305.

52. Mitchell T, Kumar P, Reddy T, et al. Dietary oxalate and kidney stone formation. *Am J Physiol Renal Physiol*. 2019;316(3):F409-F413. doi:10.1152/ajprenal.00373.2018.

53. Leffmann H. "DEATH FROM RHUBARB LEAVES DUE TO OXALIC ACID POISONING". *JAMA*. 1919;73(12):928–929. doi:10.1001/jama.1919.02610380054023

54. Sanz P, Reig R. Clinical and pathological findings in fatal plant oxalosis. A review. Am J Forensic Med Pathol. 1992 Dec;13(4):342-5. doi: 10.1097/00000433-199212000-00016. PMID: 1288268.

55. Farré M, Xirgu J, Salgado A, Peracaula R, Reig R, Sanz P. Fatal oxalic acid poisoning from sorrel soup. *Lancet*. 1989;2(8678-8679):1524. doi:10.1016/s0140-6736(89)92967-x

56. Aktas G, Alcelik A, Yalcin A, et al. Treatment of iron deficiency anemia induces weight loss and improves metabolic parameters. La Clinica Terapeutica. 2014 Mar-Apr;165(2):e87-9. DOI: 10.7471/ct.2014.1688.

57. Solati Z, Jazayeri S, Tehrani-Doost M, Mahmoodianfard S, Gohari MR. Zinc monotherapy increases serum brain-derived

neurotrophic factor (BDNF) levels and decreases depressive symptoms in overweight or obese subjects: a double-blind, randomized, placebo-controlled trial. Nutr Neurosci. 2015 May;18(4):162-8. doi: 10.1179/1476830513Y.0000000105. Epub 2014 Jan 7. PMID: 24621065.

58.   Moore E, Mander A, Ames D, Carne R, Sanders K, Watters D. Cognitive impairment and vitamin B12: a review. Int Psychogeriatr. 2012 Apr;24(4):541-56. doi: 10.1017/S1041610211002511. Epub 2012 Jan 6. PMID: 22221769.

59.   Sean P. Kane, PharmD. "Metformin Hydrochloride." *Metformin Hydrochloride - Drug Usage Statistics, ClinCalc DrugStats Database*, clincalc.com/DrugStats/Drugs/MetforminHydrochloride.

60.   Sørensen A, Mayntz D, Raubenheimer D, Simpson SJ. Protein-leverage in mice: the geometry of macronutrient balancing and consequences for fat deposition. *Obesity (Silver Spring)*. 2008;16(3): 566-571. doi:10.1038/oby.2007.58.

61.   "U.S. Food-Away-from-Home Spending Continued to Outpace Food-at-Home Spending in 2019." *USDA ERS - Chart Detail*, www.ers.usda.gov/data-products/chart-gallery/gallery/chart-detail/?chartId=58364.

Chapter 8: Getting Started

1.   Hassan AA, Sandanger TM, Brustad M. Level of selected nutrients in meat, liver, tallow and bone marrow from semi-domesticated reindeer (Rangifer t. tarandus L.). *Int J Circumpolar Health*. 2012;71:17997. Published 2012 Mar 19. doi:10.3402/ijch. v71i0.17997.

2.   Biel W, Czerniawska-Piątkowska E, Kowalczyk A. Offal Chemical Composition from Veal, Beef, and Lamb Maintained in Organic Production Systems. *Animals (Basel)*. 2019;9(8):489. Published 2019 Jul 26. doi:10.3390/ani9080489.

3.   "Statistics About Diabetes." *Statistics About Diabetes | ADA*, 22 Mar. 2018, www.diabetes.org/resources/statistics/statistics-about-diabetes.

4.   Cell Press. "How Humans Make Up For An 'Inborn' Vitamin C Deficiency." ScienceDaily. ScienceDaily, 21 March 2008. www.sciencedaily.com/releases/2008/03/080320120726.htm

5.   RODGERS, DIANA WOLF ROBB. *SACRED COW*. BENBELLA Books, 2020.

6. Williams AC, Hill LJ. Meat and Nicotinamide: A Causal Role in Human Evolution, History, and Demographics. *Int J Tryptophan Res*. 2017;10:1178646917704661. Published 2017 May 2. doi:10.1177/1178646917704661.

7. Nencioni A, Caffa I, Cortellino S, Longo VD. Fasting and cancer: molecular mechanisms and clinical application. *Nat Rev Cancer*. 2018;18(11):707-719. doi:10.1038/s41568-018-0061-0.

Chapter 9: See How She Runs

1. Peters SJ, Leblanc PJ. Metabolic aspects of low carbohydrate diets and exercise. *Nutr Metab (Lond)*. 2004;1(1):7. Published 2004 Sep 30. doi:10.1186/1743-7075-1-7.

2. Purdom, T., Kravitz, L., Dokladny, K. *et al*. Understanding the factors that effect maximal fat oxidation. *J Int Soc Sports Nutr* 15, 3 (2018). https://doi.org/10.1186/s12970-018-0207-1

3. Richter EA, Hargreaves M. Exercise, GLUT4, and skeletal muscle glucose uptake. Physiol Rev. 2013 Jul;93(3):993-1017. doi: 10.1152/physrev.00038.2012. PMID: 23899560.

4. Goyaram V, Kohn TA, Ojuka EO. Suppression of the GLUT4 adaptive response to exercise in fructose-fed rats. *Am J Physiol Endocrinol Metab*. 2014;306(3):E275-E283. doi:10.1152/ajpendo.00342.2013.

5. Lê KA, Faeh D, Stettler R, Debard C, Loizon E, Vidal H, Boesch C, Ravussin E, Tappy L. Effects of four-week high-fructose diet on gene expression in skeletal muscle of healthy men. Diabetes Metab. 2008 Feb;34(1):82-5. doi:10.1016/j.diabet.2007.08.004. Epub 2007 Dec 11. PMID: 18063403.

6. Pfeiffer B, Stellingwerff T, Hodgson AB, Randell R, Pöttgen K, Res P, Jeukendrup AE. Nutritional intake and gastrointestinal problems during competitive endurance events. Med Sci Sports Exerc. 2012 Feb;44(2):344-51. doi: 10.1249/MSS.0b013e31822dc809. PMID: 21775906.

7. Wilson PB. Dietary and non-dietary correlates of gastrointestinal distress during the cycle and run of a triathlon. Eur J Sport Sci. 2016;16(4):448-54. doi: 10.1080/17461391.2015.1046191. Epub 2015 Jul 29. PMID: 26222930.

8. Stuempfle KJ, Hoffman MD, Hew-Butler T. Association of gastrointestinal distress in ultramarathoners with race diet. Int J Sport Nutr Exerc Metab. 2013 Apr;23(2):103-9. doi: 10.1123/ijsnem.23.2.103. Epub 2012 Sep 19. PMID: 23006626